WINCHAN99

W9-CPB-305

DATE DUE

The Contraceptive Handbook

The Contraceptive Handbook.

AVAVAVAVAVAVAVAVAVAVAVAVAVAVAVAVAVAVAVAVAVAVAVAVAVAVA

A Guide to Safe and Effective Choices

Beverly Winikoff, M.D., M.P.H.
Suzanne Wymelenberg

and the Editors of
Consumer Reports Books

Consumer Reports Books
A Division of Consumers Union
Yonkers, New York

613.9
WIN

I. Title

Illustrations on pages 46 and 47 from *The Cervical Cap Handbook,* Emma Goldman Clinic, Iowa City, Iowa, 1988. Courtesy of the Emma Goldman Clinic.
Illustration on page 159 courtesy *Journal of Urology,* vol. 145, February 1991.

Library of Congress Cataloging-in-Publication Data
Winikoff, Beverly.
    The contraceptive handbook : a guide to safe and effective choices / Beverly Winikoff, Suzanne Wymelenberg, and the editors of Consumer Reports Books.
        p. cm.
    Includes bibliographical references (p.   ) and index.
    ISBN 0-89043-430-1
    1. Contraceptives—Handbooks, manuals, etc.   I. Wymelenberg, Suzanne.   II. Consumer Reports Books.   III. Title.
RG137.W56   1992
613.9'4—dc20   92-98
                                                                                        CIP

Design by Susan Hood
Drawings by Harriet Greenfield
First printing, May 1992
Manufactured in the United States of America

The Contraceptive Handbook is a Consumer Reports Book published by Consumers Union, the nonprofit organization that publishes *Consumer Reports,* the monthly magazine of test reports, product Ratings, and buying guidance. Established in 1936, Consumers Union is chartered under the Not-for-Profit Corporation Law of the State of New York.

The purposes of Consumers Union, as stated in its charter, are to provide consumers with information and counsel on consumer goods and services, to give information on all matters relating to the expenditure of the family income, and to initiate and to cooperate with individual and group efforts seeking to create and maintain decent living standards.

Contents

Acknowledgments

Many people contributed their experience and knowledge to this book as researchers, providers, or users of contraceptives. They have our warmest gratitude.

For their patience in answering our many questions, for reading part of the text and making suggestions, we are grateful to Pat Anderson, Diane Finnerty, Marc Goldstein, Betty Gonzales, Carol Lynch, Catherine Myers, Cate Nicholas, Eleanor Tabeek, Elizabeth Segal, Irving Sivin, Susan Tew, and Sandra Waldman.

For expanding our knowledge on particular issues, we thank John Fishburne, Gary Grubb, Theodore Jackanicz, Lisa Kaeser, Andrew Kaunitz, Veronica Ryback, Liz Summerhayes, and Albert Yuzpe.

Introduction

Contraception, in one form or another, has been practiced by the human community for thousands of years. Before the development of modern methods, women placed oil or honey in their vaginas or inserted sea sponges soaked in lemon juice to act as barriers to conception. Douches were a popular, if not very effective, method of birth control for women, and men had the option of using condoms, which were first used in the sixteenth century.

Today men and women want contraceptives that are safe, effective, affordable, and convenient to use. In addition, they want a varied selection of available contraceptives to accommodate changes in their life-styles. A method that is useful for spacing pregnancies is not necessarily acceptable for the woman who does not want any more children. A contraceptive that is effective for someone who has sexual intercourse infrequently may not work for young married adults.

CONTRACEPTIVE CHOICES IN THE UNITED STATES

Various methods of birth control are available in the United States today, from natural methods to condoms, the sponge,

1

spermicidal foams and jellies, diaphragms and cervical caps, the Pill, IUDs, and implants. Although none of these methods are absolutely guaranteed to protect a woman against pregnancy, they are generally quite effective if used carefully according to instructions and for every act of sexual intercourse.

There is need for improvement in the types of contraceptives available, but the United States no longer leads the world in the development of safer and surer birth control techniques. In fact, only one major pharmaceutical company in the United States today is engaged in contraceptive research and development. This situation must change if more reliable forms of birth control are to be offered to the population in the future.

CONTRACEPTIVES AND SEXUALLY TRANSMITTED DISEASES

Some contraceptives have an important use beyond birth control—they can also act as a defense against some sexually transmitted diseases (STDs). STDs can undermine your health and fertility and be passed on to a fetus. Sexually transmitted diseases also may lead to pelvic inflammatory disease, or PID, which has become epidemic in the United States. PID occurs most often when sexually transmitted bacteria travel upward from the vagina to the uterus and fallopian tubes. It also can occur after childbirth or abortion. The infection leaves behind scar tissue that may cause infertility or an ectopic pregnancy. If caught early, PID can be treated with antibiotics; if neglected, the disease can lead to chronic pain, major surgery, or even death.

At least 24 different STDs have been identified, including syphilis, gonorrhea, AIDS, genital warts, chlamydia, cytomegalovirus infections, herpes simplex, and hepatitis B. The agents that cause these diseases can be carried in semen, blood, and other body secretions.

A woman does not need to have frequent intercourse with

an infected partner in order to become infected with an STD. Medical scientists report that she has a 50 percent chance of getting gonorrhea from having intercourse just once with an infected man. A man has a 25 percent chance of acquiring gonorrhea after one act of intercourse with an infected woman. Given these statistics, the use of a barrier-type contraceptive during sexual intercourse is vital, especially with occasional or short-term relationships.

Only some types of contraceptives provide effective protection against STDs and PID. The barrier methods—the condom, the diaphragm, the cervical cap, and the contraceptive sponge—appear to be adequate, although not perfect, forms of protection.

Generally, except for barrier contraceptives, the only protection against these infections is abstinence from sexual intercourse or a long-term, mutually exclusive relationship between uninfected partners.

ABOUT THIS BOOK

The Contraceptive Handbook is a detailed guide to the methods of birth control currently available in the United States, together with an overview of new methods that are currently in development. Each chapter describes and discusses a specific device or treatment and provides the information needed to make the best choice for a particular situation. Discussions include a description of each contraceptive, its advantages and disadvantages, safety concerns, general effectiveness, side effects, costs, and how to obtain and use it. Because costs vary, a range of prices is provided for most products.

Men and women reviewing their contraceptive options should be aware that no single method of birth control is ideal or totally reliable. In addition, almost all contraceptive products have some side effects; others require a certain amount of care in their use. Choosing the right type of birth control requires carefully weighing the advantages and disadvantages of each method and keeping in mind the long-term effects, as well as the benefits and risks involved.

This book is addressed to concerned men and women of all ages who are sexually active or about to become so and who want to act responsibly in this most vital area of their lives.

1

The Anatomy and Physiology of Sex and Reproduction

A number of different methods of birth control are on the market today in the United States. In order to understand them and to decide which method is best for you, you need to know something about the male and female reproductive systems and the process of conception. This chapter outlines the anatomy and function of the male and female reproductive systems. You can refer to it easily as you read the rest of the book. You can also use this chapter to check out sexual structures that you can see and touch on your own body.

THE MALE

The sexual organs of a man consist of the testicles, the scrotum, the epididymis, the vas deferens, the prostate, the urethra, and the penis (see Figure 1.1).

The *scrotum* is the pouch of skin that hangs behind the penis and holds the testicles. It is sensitive to sexual stimulation and to changes in temperature outside the body. The scrotum's function is to keep the testicles at just the right temperature for producing sperm. It sometimes holds the testicles tight against the body to keep them warm, and at other times the scrotal sac is very loose, to allow the testicles to cool off.

The *testicles,* or *testes,* are composed of delicate, tiny, tightly coiled tubes that are lined with cells that manufacture either sperm or hormones. During the teen years, these tubes—and the testicles themselves—grow, and certain of their cells begin to secrete androgens, the male hormones (such as testosterone) that cause the body to develop such male characteristics as body and facial hair. The androgens, in turn, stimulate another type of cell in the tubes to make sperm. After puberty and until some time in old age, the continuous secretion of androgens results in a constant production of sperm.

After sperm have been made, they move into the *epididymis,* a tube that coils along the back of each testicle, where they grow. The mature sperm is composed of an oval head that contains genetic material and a long, whiplike tail that propels it with great vigor and speed. It takes a sperm approximately 72 days to grow from its earliest stage to maturity. Not all sperm mature; some die in the epididymis. When sperm are mature, they pass from the epididymis into the *vas deferens,* also known as the sperm duct. Each vas runs from the epididymis up to the outside of the bladder. As it approaches the bladder, the duct widens in order to have enough space to store sperm in preparation for an ejaculation.

Just beneath the bladder lies the *prostate* gland, which produces secretions that help sperm survive. The *urethra,* the tube that carriers urine from the bladder, passes through the prostate. The prostate secretions enter the urethra through tiny ducts and mix with the sperm just before ejaculation. This mixture of sperm and gland secretions is called *semen,* or ejaculate, and contains millions of sperm.

The male urethra has two functions. When a man urinates, it transports urine from the bladder. When he is sexually stimulated, a valve closes the opening between the bladder and the urethra to prevent urine from mixing with the semen. (Consequently, it takes a while before a man is able to urinate after becoming sexually aroused.) At the peak of sexual

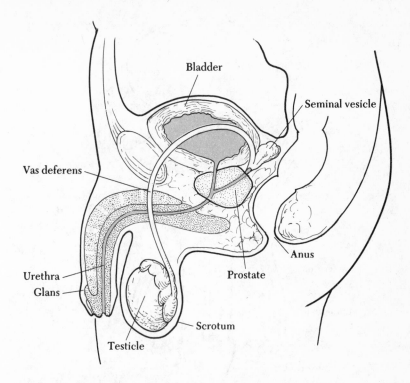

Figure 1.1 The Male Reproductive System (Side View)

excitement, muscles around the epididymis, the prostate gland, and the *seminal vesicles* contract rhythmically, forcing semen down the urethra and out the penis. This is called an orgasm, ejaculating, or having a climax. Although each ejaculate has tens of millions of sperm, only one sperm actually fertilizes an egg.

The *penis* is composed mostly of soft spongy tissue packed with a network of tiny blood vessels. Two sections of this tissue lie side by side along the upper part of the penis and help anchor it to the pubic bones. A third section lies underneath the entire length of the penis. At the tip this section broadens and forms the *glans;* at the base of the penis, it forms the bulb. The urethra enters the penis at the bulb end and opens at the glans. The penis is covered with loose skin; in addition, on an

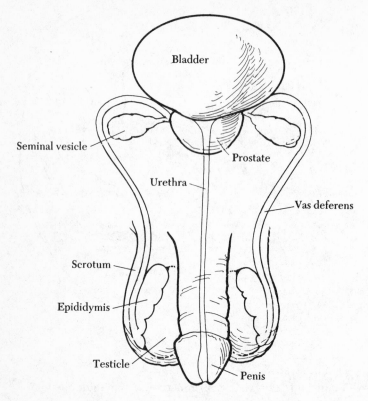

Figure 1.2 The Male Reproductive System (Front View)

uncircumcised penis, a fold of this skin, the foreskin, hangs over the glans. When a man is aroused sexually, the valve system in the blood vessels of the penis closes the usual exits in the blood network. As a result, the spongy tissues fill with blood so the penis becomes hard and erect, allowing it to penetrate the vagina.

THE FEMALE

The exterior sexual organs of the female are the mons pubis, the labia or lips of the vagina, the clitoris, the hymen, and the vaginal opening. The visible exterior sexual structures together are called the vulva or external genitalia. The vagina leads to the internal organs: the cervix, the uterus, the fallopian tubes, and the ovaries. They are inside the pelvis, supported and protected by the pelvic muscles and bones.

If you are not familiar with your sexual anatomy, especially the interior organs, looking at the following illustration is helpful, but looking at and feeling your own anatomy is a better approach. Being familiar with your own body makes it easier to use birth control and may increase your pleasure during sex. It is useful, for instance, to know the length and width of the vaginal canal and just where the cervix is located up near its end.

The *mons pubis* is the most noticeable part of the female genital area. It is the soft mound of fatty tissue below the belly that covers and protects the joining of the pubic bones, which is called the pubic symphysis. During puberty, the mons

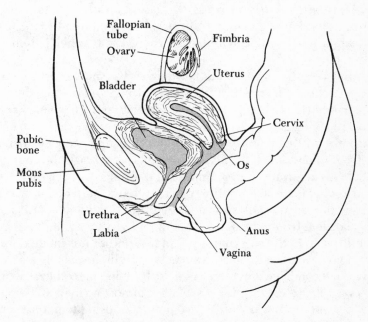

Figure 1.3 The Female Reproductive System (Side View)

becomes covered with hair, which also may grow back outside the labia majora toward the anus, the opening of the
rectum.

The opening to the vagina is protected by the *labia*. In some
women, the *labia majora*, the outermost lips around the
opening to the vagina, are darker than the surrounding skin.
The *labia minora* lie within the labia majora and are more delicate. They are sensitive to touch, and with sexual stimulation
they become filled with blood and turn darker. The area of
skin between the labia and the anus is the *perineum*, which
often is also sensitive to stimulation.

The labia minora are joined at the front to form a soft fold
of skin that looks like a little hood. This protects the *clitoris*,
the most sensitive part of the genitalia. There are many
nerves in the clitoral area, and during sexual excitement they
transmit sensory messages. The clitoris has often been compared to the penis in its anatomy and reaction to stimulation.
When a woman is aroused, her clitoris becomes erect and
very sensitive. If you press the clitoris with your fingers,
under its skin you can feel a firm but movable shaft that connects it to the pubic symphysis, where the two pelvic bones
meet.

Between the clitoris and the vagina is the small aperture for
the *urethra*. The urethra transports urine from the bladder.

In addition to being shielded by the labia, the *vaginal opening* in young girls may be partially covered by the *hymen*. This
usually stretchable, thin tissue is partially open and lets menstrual blood pass through. Frequently, when intercourse
takes place for the first time, the opening in the hymen is
stretched further. Sometimes it is pushed so hard that it tears,
so it bleeds and hurts for a short time. The hymen varies a
great deal from woman to woman and girl to girl in its flexibility and in the size of its opening. Whether it is intact does
not always indicate that a woman is a virgin. A sexually active
woman can have a hymen that is still in one piece because it
is very flexible. Or a virgin may have almost no hymen. Being
a virgin does not prevent a woman from using tampons, for
example.

The *vagina* is the passage that connects the cervix to the external genitalia. Its length varies from 2½ to 4 inches. It has muscular walls that are lined with a mucous membrane and contain many blood vessels. When examined with the fingers, the vagina feels soft and muscular. In most women, the lower third is sensitive to sexual stimulation and the upper portion is less responsive. The vagina's walls are folded in on themselves so closely they touch, yet they have a great capacity for expanding during sexual excitement and for stretching and fitting around an object such as a penis, a baby, or a diaphragm. Its mucous membrane can change from almost dry to very wet. It secretes fluids, particularly around the time of ovulation, during pregnancy, and when the woman is sexually aroused. The vagina slants back slightly toward the spine. It is connected to the uterus just above its neck, the cervix.

Resembling an upside-down pear, the *uterus* is approximately the size of a fist and has thick, muscular walls. The lower, narrow end of the uterus is called the *cervix*. The cervix extends down into the vagina, where it has an opening

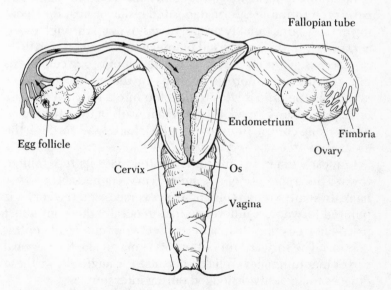

Figure 1.4 The Female Reproductive System (Front View)

called the *os*. The cervix is small and firm and feels like the tip
of the nose. Before a woman has a child, the os is very small,
about the diameter of a straw. The cervix and uterus have
great flexibility so they can accommodate pregnancy and
childbirth. Afterward they usually remain somewhat larger.
Glands in the cervix secrete mucus that varies in amount and
consistency during the month, depending on the levels of
estrogen or progesterone, hormones produced by the woman's body. When progesterone levels are high, the cervix
secretes a thick, nonstretchable mucus that effectively plugs
the os against sperm; in contrast, during ovulation, high levels
of estrogen cause a thin, stretchy mucus that is receptive to
sperm.

On some days the cervix is easier to reach than on others
because it shifts position during the menstrual cycle. Just
before menstruation the cervix is lower in the vagina, and a
few days before ovulation it pulls up. The os also changes
throughout the cycle, opening wider before ovulation and
before menstruation.

If nothing blocks their way and the mucus in the vagina and
cervix is hospitable, sperm deposited inside or near the opening of the vagina quickly propel themselves up through the os
and then into the uterus and fallopian tubes, where fertilization occurs. After fertilization, the developing egg cell moves
into the uterus, where it implants in the *endometrium*, or
uterine lining, and begins to develop into a fetus. When the
fetus is fully developed, the muscular walls of the uterus produce strong contractions to push the infant down through the
greatly enlarged os and vagina.

In most women the uterus is slanted, with its top pointed
toward the upper abdomen and the cervix aimed at the lower
back. In some women this angle is reversed, and the cervix is
pointed forward, a difference that generally does not affect
pregnancy or childbirth but can affect your choice of contraception. The forward tilt of the cervix may make the cervical
cap or diaphragm less reliable because the angle allows these
devices to be easily dislodged during intercourse.

On each side of the uterus is an *ovary* and a *fallopian tube*, also known as an oviduct or egg tube. The ovaries are small, oval shaped, and about the size of walnuts. They contain thousands of tiny egg follicles that hold a lifetime supply of undeveloped egg cells. They also produce certain hormones needed for reproduction. Each ovary is adjacent to a slender, delicate fallopian tube, which is about 4 inches long. The end of each tube is shaped somewhat like a funnel with fringed ends, called the fimbria, that almost touch the ovaries. When an egg matures and is pushed out of the ovary, the fimbria gather it up into the fallopian tube (see Figure 1.4). The egg is moved slowly down the fallopian tube to the uterus.

Ovulation

At the time a baby girl is born, her two ovaries contain all the egg cells, or oocytes, needed for ovulation during her entire lifetime. Of the million or so oocytes that have the potential to develop into eggs during a woman's reproductive years between puberty and menopause, only about 300 to 500 actually will be ovulated. As a girl matures, her body steps up the production of the hormones that affect ovulation and reproduction. The most important hormones are estrogen, progesterone, follicle-stimulating hormone (FSH), luteinizing hormone (LH), and gonadotropin-releasing hormone (GnRH).

The production of each of these hormones increases and decreases in a regular pattern every month. During this cycle, changes in hormone levels cause one (rarely two or more) egg in an ovary to mature and then be expelled. Each egg develops within a follicle, a hollow sphere of cells. When the egg is ready for fertilization, the follicle breaks open, the egg floats out, and it is captured by the fimbria. Usually only one egg cell develops each month; if two eggs mature and both are fertilized successfully, the result is fraternal twins. (Identical twins result when one fertilized egg splits in two.)

While the egg is maturing, increased levels of other hormones cause the lining of the uterus to thicken and soften, in preparation for nurturing a fertilized egg.

The menstrual cycle begins with the first day of menstruation, which is termed day one. Ovulation usually takes place approximately halfway between menstrual periods, most often 14 days before the next menstrual period (see Chapter 13).

Physical and emotional events in a woman's life can have a considerable effect on hormone production. Changes in hormone levels can alter the menstrual cycle; as a result, ovulation can occur at an unexpected time. In rare instances ovulation has been known to take place even during menstruation.

A sperm can live in the fallopian tubes for two or three days, and an egg cell can be fertilized up to 24 hours after it leaves the ovary. Therefore, a woman may be fertile for a minimum of three to four days during each menstrual cycle. (It is not known precisely how long eggs and sperm live in the human reproductive system; for the best protection against pregnancy, use a contraceptive before every act of intercourse.) If an egg is unfertilized, it is simply absorbed by the uterus or flushed out with the menstrual blood.

Fertilization

To be fertilized successfully, the egg must be penetrated by a single sperm not long after ovulation. Although each ejaculation contains millions of sperm, only a few hundred usually reach the fallopian tubes, a journey that takes healthy sperm about 30 minutes. If ovulation has just occurred, the sperm will encounter an egg cell ready for fertilization. The egg cell is covered by a thick, tough, translucent layer called the zona pellucida, which functions as a sophisticated biological security system that chemically controls the entry of sperm into the egg. Although there may be hundreds of tail-lashing sperm clustered around the egg itself, only one, perhaps the most vigorous, actually succeeds in penetrating the zona pellucida. As soon as it does, a chemical reaction shuts out the rest. This reaction prevents the genetic confusion that would occur if the genes of more than one sperm combined with the genes of the egg.

When an egg is fertilized, the genetic material from the sperm and egg merges, and the egg cell begins to divide. It takes approximately three or four days for a fertilized egg to move through the fallopian tubes and enter the uterus. During that time it has about a 50 percent chance of failing to develop further. If it survives, it continues to divide, and by the time it reaches the uterus it is a cluster of cells the size of a speck of dust. By the sixth or seventh day after ovulation, the cluster begins to embed itself in the endometrium, the lining of the uterus, which has become thick, soft, and engorged with blood in preparation for nurturing an embryo. The cells continue to divide, and by the eighteenth day after fertilization, the first cells that eventually will form the spinal cord can be detected. At this point the cluster of cells can be called a true embryo.

Tubal Pregnancy

If the fallopian tube is abnormal in some way or damaged from pelvic inflammatory disease, the fertilized egg may not be able to reach the uterus. Instead it begins to grow in the fallopian tube. Such a pregnancy is called tubal, or ectopic. As the embryo grows, it frequently ruptures or damages the fallopian tube and the structures around it. Tubal pregnancies can be life-threatening. The symptoms include abdominal pain and vaginal bleeding. Treatment consists of surgery to remove the embryo tissue and repair damaged structures. About one in 100 pregnancies in the United States today is ectopic.

Menstruation

If fertilization does not take place and no cell cluster is implanted in the endometrium, the production of certain hormones declines, and the blood-filled endometrium, no longer needed to nourish an embryo, breaks up. Over several days, it is expelled from the uterus, sometimes with the help of contractions that may range from mild to painful. This shedding of tissue and blood is called menstruation, or a period.

This cycle of events occurs every month unless an egg is fertilized and successfully attaches to the uterine lining. When attachment occurs, the lining is not expelled, there is no menstrual bleeding, and a pregnancy is under way.

SEXUAL INTERCOURSE

When a woman becomes sexually aroused, a cascade of changes occur through her body. Blood flow to the genital area increases, and her clitoris swells, becomes erect, and is extremely sensitive. The labia minora swell and deepen in color, and the vagina becomes moist. Its opening widens, and the upper part of the vagina itself expands to almost twice its size. The lower section tightens. All the genital area seems to increase in sensitivity. The breasts enlarge and the nipples become erect. The woman's heart rate speeds up, she breathes faster and harder, and all her muscles tighten. If sexual stimulation continues, particularly of the clitoris, arousal intensifies and leads to an orgasm. During orgasm, the muscles around the vagina, uterus, and rectum contract once or several times and then release.

If lovemaking doesn't continue, the process slowly begins to reverse. Muscles relax, blood flows out of the swollen tissues, and the clitoris and vagina return to their usual size.

When a man is sexually stimulated, his body undergoes many of the same physical changes. The penis becomes erect as blood flows into the spongy tissues, while a system of valves closes vessel exits so the tissues fill with blood. Muscles in the pelvis tighten and force semen from the prostate and epididymis into the urethra. If sexual stimulation continues, it affects the spinal nerves, which in turn propel the semen through the urethra and out the penis. A valve at the base of the bladder closes during this process to prevent ejaculate from entering the bladder. It also prevents urine from mixing with the semen. Afterward, the muscles relax, the valves in the penile blood system open, the blood quickly drains away, and the penis becomes soft again.

After orgasm, most men experience a period during which they have no physical response to further sexual stimulation. Many women don't appear to go through this period, and some women, if stimulation continues, can experience multiple orgasms.

HOW CONTRACEPTION WORKS

The various methods of birth control function at different points in the reproductive process. They either stop the sperm and the egg from meeting in the fallopian tube, suppress ovulation, or create an environment hostile to fertilization and implantation.

- Barrier contraceptives such as the condom, the diaphragm, the cervical cap, and the contraceptive sponge physically block sperm from entering the cervix.
- A chemical spermicide in creams, jellies, foams, sponges, vaginal suppositories, and pieces of film kills sperm when they enter the vagina.
- Birth control pills and Norplant implants slightly alter the normal hormone levels in women. The combined pill suppresses ovulation by supplying the body with small, extra amounts of synthetic versions of the female hormones estrogen and progesterone. Progestin-only pills and Norplant also suppress ovulation but not consistently. They also thicken the cervical mucus to make it impregnable to sperm, and they hinder the normal monthly changes in the lining of the uterus.
- Intrauterine devices (IUDs) change the environment of the fallopian tubes to make them inhospitable to sperm and eggs and prevent fertilization.
- Sterilization is surgery to block the woman's fallopian tubes or the man's vasa deferentia. It is highly effective and the most commonly used method in the United States.
- Fertility awareness methods teach a woman how to

know when she is fertile. During those days she and her partner either abstain from intercourse or use a barrier contraceptive.

- If an egg has been fertilized, morning-after contraception can prevent implantation. If it already has implanted (six or seven days after fertilization), the pregnancy can be terminated with an abortion.

One

ᴧᴠᴧ

Barrier Methods

2

The Condom

The condom is a soft sheath that fits over the penis. It is made of rubber latex or treated animal tissue that is very thin, strong, and flexible. Because a condom prevents seminal fluid from entering the vagina, it is a very effective barrier to conception. It also protects both partners from the organisms that cause such STDs as syphilis, AIDS, gonorrhea, trichomoniasis, candidiasis, chlamydia, genital warts, and cytomegalovirus.

Most condoms measure between 7 and 8 inches long and are approximately 2 inches in diameter. Because there is little variation in the size of men's erect penises, an exact fit is not important. Thus condoms are not sold by size. (The terms "large" and "small" on the package refer to the size of the package and the number of condoms in it, not the size of the condom.) The open end of the condom has a rubber ring that makes it easier to put on and take off; the ring also helps to keep the condom in place. Sometimes the closed end is made with a small extra pouch, or reservoir, for the semen.)

Condoms, or "rubbers," are easy to use, don't cost very much, and don't require a physical examination or a doctor's prescription. Moreover, they are available in small packets and can be tucked into a pocket or purse or stored in a bedside table or bathroom cabinet.

Condoms are available in dozens of brands and models, ranging from plain to those that come in a variety of thicknesses, colors, printed designs, and textures, with or without a lubricant or spermicide. Both latex and "skin" condoms come in several shapes: tapered, flared, or contoured for a tighter fit. The choice of a shape is entirely personal; it doesn't affect condom wear, although a condom with a reservoir tip may be less likely to break or leak when filled with semen.

CONDOMS AND SEXUAL PLEASURE

Although some men complain that wearing a condom slightly diminishes their pleasure, half the 2,500 men who responded to a survey published in the March 1989 issue of *Consumer Reports* said they liked condoms because the small decrease in stimulation allowed them to prolong sexual play. This seldom-mentioned aspect of condoms is particularly useful for the man who is easily aroused or ejaculates prematurely.

Skin condoms made from treated lamb membrane are preferred by some users because they are thinner than the latex ones. (However, they do not protect against the AIDS virus.) Thinner latex condoms may also permit more stimulation, although they can tear more easily than regular latex condoms. Some men are unable to enjoy intercourse or maintain an erection while wearing a condom, regardless of the type used.

Many women especially like the condom. It's an effective method of birth control that has no side effects and protects them against sexually transmitted diseases, including AIDS. Condoms also can be used during pregnancy, as a protection against diseases that might affect the fetus.

Almost half the condoms sold today are bought by women. Instead of viewing the condom as an unwelcome interruption, many women and men have made the act of sheathing the penis a part of their lovemaking. A survey of condom users found that it is often sexually stimulating for both partners when the woman puts the condom on the penis.

LATEX VERSUS SKIN CONDOMS

Although most condoms are made of latex, skin condoms are also available. Made from part of a lamb's large intestine, they are stronger than the rubber varieties. Some men and women find that they feel more sensation with this type. Skin condoms are slightly more porous than latex condoms. This porosity does not affect their ability to prevent pregnancy—sperm are larger than the pores—but such organisms as the AIDS and hepatitis B viruses can pass through. Therefore, the Food and Drug Administration (FDA) does not allow skin condoms to be labeled as protection against sexually transmitted diseases. If protection against infection is an important concern, latex condoms are considered the better choice. Skin condoms are also more expensive than latex condoms.

Extra-thin latex condoms permit more sensation, but they also tear more easily than regular latex condoms and must be handled carefully.

Latex condoms are available with dry lubrication that usually has a silicone base; others are lubricated with a water-based surgical jelly. Condoms also are available with a coating that contains the spermicide nonoxynol-9; however, the amount of this active ingredient varies from one type of condom to another and is not a substitute for a vaginal spermicide.

EFFECTIVENESS

The failure rate for condoms ranges from 4 percent to 14 percent, or 4 to 14 pregnancies among every 100 women during the first year of using this method of birth control. (With most contraceptives, the greatest number of failures occurs during the first year of use.) Condoms fail for two reasons: because of human error or because the product itself had a flaw. A condom is an effective contraceptive only if you use a new one with each act of intercourse and if you use it correctly—rolled all the way on and removed carefully. Condoms can break because of a weakness in the rubber, but such breakage rarely happens. Most condom failures are the result of human error.

The FDA routinely checks various brands of condoms by filling randomly selected samples with water to see whether they leak or develop bulges that indicate a weak spot in the rubber. A better test is to inflate the condom with air. The greatest pressure and volume of air that a condom can withstand before it bursts is then recorded. (Don't test a condom yourself by filling it beforehand with water or air. Doing so will only weaken it.)

HEALTH EFFECTS

Condoms may produce an allergic reaction in either partner. The reaction may be caused by the spermicidal coating or by the latex or lamb "skin" itself. Sometimes perfume or the amount of nonoxynol-9 in a particular spermicide causes a reaction, and switching to another type of condom or spermicide solves the problem. If that approach is not successful, then the spermicide should be eliminated as the possible cause of the reaction; that is, the man should use nonspermicidal condoms for a couple of weeks, and the woman should not use spermicidal foams or creams. The best time to do this

WHO SHOULDN'T USE CONDOMS?

Condoms are not the best birth control method (1) if you tend to forget to keep a supply of condoms on hand, (2) if you are inclined to skip using protection "just this once," or (3) if you or your partner are embarrassed or uncomfortable using condoms. And if a condom substantially reduces your pleasure despite trying to incorporate it into your lovemaking, you also should find a different contraceptive method.

test is during the safer part of the menstrual cycle—just before, during, or immediately after menstruation. If the irritation persists, the latex may be the problem. Try other brands of latex or skin condoms, keeping in mind that the latter do not protect you against AIDS.

USING A CONDOM

If condoms are new to you, read the package instructions carefully. Also, it's not a bad idea to practice putting one on. You can practice on your own erect penis as well as on cylinder-shaped objects or vegetables. (Discard the practice condom.)

A condom comes rolled up in a package, so it must be unrolled all the way up the erect penis. If you are not circumcised, pull back the foreskin before putting on the condom. If the condom doesn't have a reservoir tip, grasp about half an inch of its tip between two fingers as you roll it on with the other hand. This allows room for the semen and lessens the chance that the condom will be stressed and break when it's full. Also help to avoid breakage by pinching out any air at the tip. Air plus semen can exert too much pressure on the latex and tear it. As you handle the condom, be careful not to tear it with your fingernails or rings. Until the condom is securely in place, keep the penis away from the vagina—drops of semen can leak from the penis before ejaculation.

For additional protection: Before intercourse, insert into the vagina an applicator of spermicidal foam or a cream or jelly made to be used with a diaphragm. Although some condoms are pretreated with a spermicide, it may not be enough to offer adequate protection. Spermicide is especially recommended at the most fertile time in a woman's menstrual cycle (see Chapter 6).

Use a new condom every time you have intercourse. This is the most important rule in the successful use of condoms. The average man produces millions of healthy, active sperm every day, and the supply is seldom diminished by frequent ejacu-

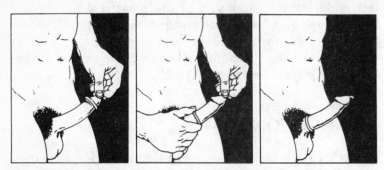

The right way to use a condom:
1. Place the rolled-up condom on the end of the erect penis. Hold the tip of the condom (about a half inch) to squeeze out the air. This leaves room for the semen to collect after ejaculation.
2. Keep holding the tip of the condom with one hand. With the other hand, unroll the condom down the length of the erect penis. (Uncircumcised men should first pull back the foreskin.)
3. Unroll the condom all the way down to the pubic hair.
4. Put the condom on before entering your partner.
5. You can use a water-based lubricant (check the label or ask a pharmacist) such as K-Y Lubricating Jelly or Today Personal Lubricant. Oil-based lubricants like mineral oil, baby oil, vegetable oil, petroleum jelly, or cold cream should *not* be used, since they can damage the condom.
6. Right after ejaculation: (a) hold onto the condom as you (b) pull out while the penis is still erect.

Figure 2.1   How to Use a Condom

lations. No matter how many times you have intercourse during a 24-hour period, use a new condom for each ejaculation.

Oils are dangerous to latex condoms. If oils or oil-based lotions touch a latex condom, its strength is reduced, and it becomes vulnerable to tearing during use and can even develop tiny holes. Keep baby oils, petroleum jelly, hand lotions, face creams, ointments, and makeup away from condoms and other latex rubber contraceptives (diaphragms, cervical caps). Wash your hands before touching a condom.

Don't begin intercourse until the vagina is well lubricated. When a woman is sexually aroused, the vagina naturally lubricates. Without this lubrication, the condom can tear. If you want more lubrication, use water, a contraceptive cream or jelly made for diaphragms, or a *water-based* lubricating jelly such as K-Y Jelly, Ortho-Gynol, Koromex Gel, or H-R Lubricating Jelly, which are sold in the feminine hygiene section of drugstores. If you're in doubt about a product, the list of ingredients on the package indicates whether it contains any oil.

After ejaculation, withdraw the penis when it is still erect, to prevent the condom from slipping off. Pull the penis slowly from the vagina while holding the condom carefully near its rim so semen doesn't spill out. Look at the condom for signs of leakage. If it's leaking or if it comes off while still in the vagina, at once insert an application of a spermicide well up into the vagina. This is not a guarantee against pregnancy or infection, but it is good protection nonetheless.

Use a condom only once. This rule is especially important for protection against sexually transmitted diseases. Before you have intercourse again, put on a new condom.

Care and Storage

Condoms last for several years if they are kept sealed in their package and stored away from light and heat. The refrigerator is a good place to keep condoms—and any other rubber contraceptive—especially in hot weather. Condoms deteriorate if kept in the glove compartment of a car, for instance, or in a purse or coat hung in a warm closet or left for a while in the sun or near a stove or radiator. Condoms can also weaken if they are exposed to body heat for some time by being carried in an inside pocket. Don't remove the condom from the package until you are ready to use it.

Cost

Prices for latex condoms range from $3 for a dozen to more than $18 a dozen. Skin condoms are more expensive—$2 or more each. Some brands of skin condoms may cost as much as $30 a dozen.

3

The Diaphragm

The diaphragm is a shallow rubber cap with a rim made of a fine, flexible spring. It fits snugly and comfortably across the upper vagina, covering the entire cervix, thus preventing sperm from getting into the uterus and fallopian tubes and fertilizing an egg. It must be used with a spermicide.

The diaphragm is a popular method of birth control because it does not cause any hormonal or chemical changes in the body. It has almost no side effects and does not necessarily have to interrupt lovemaking. When used consistently, a diaphragm plus spermicide offers quite good protection against pregnancy and sexually transmitted diseases. The risk of pelvic inflammatory disease (PID) is reduced substantially by the use of a diaphragm.

Many couples like the idea of using a contraceptive only when the woman is fertile. The diaphragm is a particularly good method if you don't have sex frequently or if you know in advance when you will have intercourse. If you own a diaphragm but are now on the Pill, the diaphragm can provide good emergency protection if you run out of pills or are vulnerable to pregnancy because you forgot to take two or more in succession. The diaphragm is also useful when you want to have intercourse during menstruation, because it temporarily blocks the flow of blood from the uterus.

The diaphragm has several disadvantages. To be most effective, it must be used with a spermicide, must be inserted within a few hours before intercourse, and must remain in place for at least six hours afterward. As a result, it must be kept handy even when you don't expect to have sex. It also means it's necessary to keep a supply of spermicide on hand at all times.

During oral sex, some creams or jellies may have an unpleasant taste. This problem usually can be solved by wiping off the clitoris and labia after inserting the diaphragm. Both flavored and unflavored creams are available.

A spermicide is necessary because the diaphragm itself is not completely effective. The vagina flexes and changes shape during intercourse. As a result, the diaphragm cannot provide

ARE YOU A GOOD CANDIDATE FOR THE DIAPHRAGM?

If spontaneous, uninterrupted sex is important to you or your partner, and stopping at any point to put in the diaphragm is a nuisance that would discourage your use of it, then consider another method of birth control. Some women wear the diaphragm every time they and their partners are together, or they put it in every night. If necessary, fresh jelly or foam can be added closer to the time of intercourse. Other couples make inserting the diaphragm a part of their lovemaking.

Using this contraceptive effectively also requires a certain amount of planning ahead so that both the diaphragm and a supply of spermicide are at hand. If you are not likely to remember to take them along when you are going to be away from home or traveling, another method is a better choice.

The diaphragm is also a good method of birth control for the woman who shouldn't use oral contraceptives for health reasons, such as heart problems, or for the woman who smokes.

a perfect seal, and some sperm may slip past it. To protect against this possibility, a spermicidal jelly or cream is used with the diaphragm. An important function of the device is to hold spermicide close to the cervical opening to destroy any sperm that get past it. Almost all spermicides contain nonoxynol-9 as the active ingredient. Approximately two teaspoons of spermicidal cream or jelly are put inside the diaphragm before it is inserted.

EFFECTIVENESS

Rates of failure vary, ranging from approximately 2 to 20 pregnancies per 100 women during the first year of use. For a typical user, someone who is not absolutely consistent in using it, the rate is more likely to be 17 to 20 percent for the first 12 months. The diaphragm's effectiveness depends directly on how carefully and consistently it is used. Using the diaphragm without a spermicide and leaving it at home are two of the most common reasons for a high failure rate.

Age and the frequency of intercourse also affect the chance of failure. Diaphragm users who are under 25 or who have intercourse often run a greater risk of becoming pregnant. Men and women in their teens and twenties usually are extremely fertile and, accordingly, are at a greater risk of pregnancy. Moreover, when intercourse is frequent, there are more chances for failure.

To prevent pregnancy, it is best to use the diaphragm *every time* you have intercourse, including during menstruation and the so-called "safe" days shortly before menstruation. The effectiveness of the diaphragm can be enhanced if the male partner also uses a condom during the most fertile days of the month (see Chapter 13).

HEALTH EFFECTS

As a rule, the diaphragm produces no serious, negative effects on the body, nor can it be lost in the vagina or in the upper reproductive tract. Diaphragms may cause one or two side effects, however.

Urinary Infections

Some women who wear diaphragms have a slightly increased risk of repeated urinary tract infections. The pressure of the rim on the urethra and bladder may be a factor. A diaphragm in a smaller size or with a different rim may cause less pressure and resolve the problem. As precautions against infection, the diaphragm should be washed thoroughly with soap after each use, and the user should wash her hands before taking it from its case.

Allergic Reactions

In some instances, a diaphragm user or her partner proves allergic to the rubber or spermicide. Women experience this problem more often than men, developing an irritation in the vagina. The cause may be a sensitivity to the perfumes used in certain spermicides or to nonoxynol-9, the active ingredient in all but one of the spermicides on the market today. Using an unscented cream or jelly, or one that contains less nonoxynol-9, may solve the problem. If the allergy appears to be caused by the rubber, however, a different method of contraception may be required. To discover if the allergy is from the spermicide, insert some by itself into the vagina without the diaphragm and without having intercourse.

Beneficial Effects

The spermicide is effective against the organisms that cause such STDs as gonorrhea, genital herpes, trichomoniasis, and syphilis. However, it may not be as effective against chlamydia. In addition, cancer of the cervix has been found to be greatly reduced in women who faithfully used a diaphragm during intercourse for at least five years.

USING THE DIAPHRAGM

Diaphragms are available from women's health clinics and Planned Parenthood clinics, from physicians, particularly family practitioners and gynecologists, and from nurse-midwives, nurse-practitioners, and other health professionals specializing in family planning. Spermicidal creams also are available from these sources or in the feminine hygiene sections of drugstores.

Types of Diaphragms

Diaphragms are available in sizes measured in millimeters, ranging from 50 to 95 millimeters (about 2 to 4 inches) in diameter. The size you need depends on the size of your upper vagina, which is related to your body size and weight. Vaginal childbirth also affects the size. Diaphragms also are available with four types of rims that make it possible to fit this contraceptive to many different bodies.

The arcing spring rim is the most popular because for many women it is the easiest to insert. Also available is a flat spring rim, which exerts a very gentle pressure. It often is the best choice for the woman whose vaginal muscles are very firm because she has not yet had a baby. A third type has a stronger coil spring rim, designed for the vagina with a more relaxed muscle wall. A fourth is an arcing spring that bends in only two places; some women find this type easier to handle.

Both the arcing spring and coil spring types are available with an extra "wide seal" inner rim of soft latex. This is intended to create a better seal with the vaginal wall and to be more effective in holding the spermicide around the opening of the cervix.

Being Fitted

Because the diaphragm must fit very well, it is necessary to have an internal examination by a physician or other health professional before being fitted. The examination rules out any problem that would prevent you from using a diaphragm successfully, such as an abnormality of the vagina, cervix, or uterus. During the exam, the practitioner will also assess which type and size of the diaphragm will fit best. This usually is done with fitting rings or sample diaphragms, and several may have to be tried to find the size that is comfortable yet fits securely in the vagina. The ideal one is the largest size that is snug without discomfort. A diaphragm is a good fit if it touches the walls of the vagina with just enough room to insert a finger.

If you are not comfortable with the idea of inserting and removing a diaphragm by hand, some diaphragms can be used with a plastic introducer or inserter. Discuss this possibility with your practitioner.

Part of the fitting procedure must include a lesson on how to insert and remove the diaphragm. You should be given plenty of opportunity to practice while you are still in the examining room. If the rim is too stiff to be squeezed together by one hand, a type with a less firm spring may be preferable. Although more practice with the diaphragm makes it easier to use, you should feel fairly comfortable about inserting it before you leave.

It is usually possible to take the diaphragm home to practice inserting it and then, while wearing it, to go back to your practitioner to make sure it's in the right place. The idea is to be able to put it in and take it out correctly and easily before you actually use it. If the diaphragm is a good fit, you should not be able to feel it. The diaphragm may not be a good fit if you feel the need to urinate shortly after you put it in or have a sense of pressure on your abdomen. When abdominal pain, back pain, or a pain down the leg accompanies use of the diaphragm, the fit should be checked. Do not accept one that causes you any discomfort when it is correctly placed.

How to Insert the Diaphragm

Before inserting the diaphragm, wash your hands. Fill the diaphragm almost two-thirds full of a spermicidal ointment (a

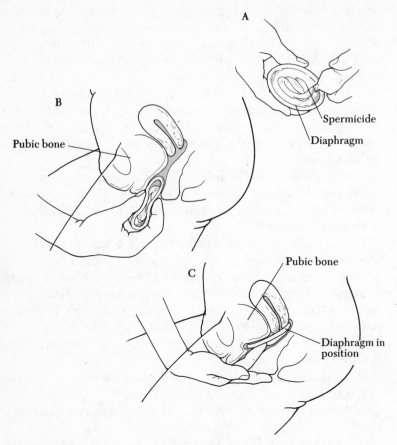

Figure 3.1 How to Insert a Diaphragm

couple of inches—about 2 to 3 teaspoons). How much you
need depends on its size: a larger diaphragm requires a little
more spermicide. Spread it all around and up on the inside of
the rim. For extra protection, some women smear a bit of the
cream on the outside of the diaphragm or put a dab on one
place on the outer rim, which is less messy. Avoid getting a
lot of cream or jelly on the outside of the rim itself; you may
create a Frisbee effect and find the diaphragm flying out of
your hand.

Some women insert the diaphragm while sitting on the toilet; others do it lying down with their legs bent or squatting. The aim is to be relaxed and comfortable.

With the open side of the cup facing upward, firmly squeeze the rim of the diaphragm together between thumb and fingers to fold it for insertion. If the spermicide has made the rim too slippery to grasp, wipe it from the outer edge but not from the inside of the diaphragm. A little spermicide in one place on the leading edge of rim helps it to slide more easily into the vagina.

While you hold the folded diaphragm in one hand with the contraceptive ointment facing up, spread apart the lips of the vagina with the other hand and then ease the diaphragm up into the vaginal canal. The leading edge of the rim should slip under and behind the cervix and lightly touch the vaginal wall. Then gently push the other edge up behind the pubic bone. When it's in the correct position, the diaphragm covers the cervix, feels comfortable, and is firmly in place.

Make sure the rim of the diaphragm is tucked up behind the pubic bone and that the cervix is covered by the soft rubber dome. This step also makes certain the contraceptive cream is in contact with the cervical opening, thoroughly protecting the cervix and uterus from sperm.

If the diaphragm feels uncomfortable, it's not correctly positioned. Take it out and try again. You may want to try a different position and make more of an effort to keep the leading edge of the diaphragm a little lower so it slips under the cervix. It usually feels awkward at first, but with practice most women become very adept at using a diaphragm.

The Spermicide

Spermicide loses its effectiveness as time passes. If you inserted the diaphragm more than two hours before intercourse, squeeze another applicator of spermicide into your vagina without disturbing the diaphragm.

To use the plastic applicator that comes with spermicidal creams or jellies, remove the cap from the tube and attach the applicator in its place. Squeeze the tube so the jelly or cream fills the applicator. Disconnect the applicator and insert it well into your vagina, just as you would a tampon, and then push the plunger in as far as it will go. When you remove the applicator, don't tug on the plunger, because that might pull some of the cream back into the applicator. Contraceptive foams, also available in most drugstores, can be used with the diaphragm instead of jelly or cream (see Chapter 6). You can apply the spermicide while still in bed or in the bathroom. It takes only a moment.

Don't use petroleum jelly or any other oil-based ointments instead of a spermicide. For one thing, they cannot kill sperm that get over the rim. Furthermore, an oil-based product can damage the rubber, allowing sperm, viruses, and bacteria to pass through. If you want to use a lubricant during intercourse, use additional spermicide or a water-based lubricant such as K-Y Jelly, Ortho-Gynol, Koromex Gel, or H-R Lubricating Jelly.

Afterward

After the last act of intercourse, leave the diaphragm in place for at least six hours. It can take that long for the spermicide to kill all the sperm. Although the diaphragm can be dislodged if the vagina flexes a great deal during intercourse, you can safely take a bath, swim, shower, bicycle, and perform almost any kind of physical activity without affecting it. You also can have a bowel movement without dislodging it.

Don't douche while wearing a diaphragm. Douching washes away protective contraceptive creams and can force sperm up into the cervix.

You can leave the diaphragm in place for longer than six hours, and many women prefer to do so. It's often more convenient to wait until morning to remove it. But to avoid the possibility of toxic shock syndrome, don't leave it in for more than 24 hours. Wear a minipad or a tampon as a shield against any jelly or sperm that may leak from the vagina after you remove the diaphragm.

Further Intercourse

Before each additional act of intercourse, add an applicator of spermicide. If six or more hours have passed and you expect to have intercourse again, you can remove and wash the diaphragm if you wish, add more jelly or cream, and reinsert it. If you are wearing the diaphragm constantly over a period of time, remove it for several hours whenever possible or occasionally ask your partner to use a condom instead.

Removing the Diaphragm

Again, wash your hands. Then find a comfortable position. Hook a finger under the part of the diaphragm rim that rests behind the pubic bone or at any other point toward the front of the vagina. Firmly pull forward and down. If it's a good fit, it may take a bit of effort to dislodge the diaphragm. Be careful not to poke a fingernail through it.

Because a certain amount of sperm and contraceptive cream comes out of the vagina with the diaphragm, many

---

DIAPHRAGM POINTERS

- Take your diaphragm with you when you go on vacation or away for the weekend. If you travel frequently, keep a second diaphragm and supply of spermicide in your travel kit.
- Always keep a tube of spermicide and its applicator with your diaphragm in its case.
- If the diaphragm becomes dislodged during intercourse, immediately add more spermicide into the vagina.
- If you are not sure that you are correctly inserting the diaphragm, or if it doesn't feel comfortable, have the placement checked by the health care provider who fitted you. Meanwhile, have your partner use a condom for extra protection. It's always a good idea to keep a supply of condoms on hand.

women remove their diaphragms while sitting on the toilet. The use of a minipad or tampon protects against any leakage afterward.

Care and Storage

Simple care of your diaphragm extends its life and effectiveness. After using it, wash it with soap and warm water, rinse, and pat it dry with a clean towel. (A diaphragm should not be put away while still wet.) Don't use antiseptics or any strong cleansing solutions on a diaphragm because they weaken the rubber. To protect it further, dust it with cornstarch. Don't use talcum powder or any perfumed powders. Store your diaphragm in its case, and don't expose it to sunlight or extreme heat.

Check your diaphragm every few weeks for holes, especially around the rim. Even the tiniest pinhole can admit hundreds of sperm. To make a check, hold it up to the light or fill it with water. The rubber in your diaphragm will gradually grow darker with time; this does not affect its function. Replace the diaphragm when the rubber shows signs of deterioration, such as cracks or brittleness.

Follow-up Care

Your diaphragm and its fit should be checked every 18 months or so. This can be done at the same time you have a pelvic exam and a Pap smear. The fit should also be checked in the following circumstances:

- if you have lost or gained more than 20 pounds
- if you've had a child, a miscarriage, an abortion, or any type of surgery involving your reproductive organs
- anytime you experience discomfort, pain, or recurring bladder infections after using the diaphragm
- anytime you suspect your diaphragm is not fitting properly or that you might not be inserting it correctly

COST

The diaphragm itself costs $12 to $25. (It is available for less from some birth control or women's health clinics, such as Planned Parenthood clinics.) The medical examination and the fitting of the diaphragm can cost from $50 to $100 or more, depending on where it is done and how extensive the examination is. The cost of the diaphragm may be included in the charge for the examination.

Prices of spermicidal jellies and creams begin at $8, and the tubes vary in size. An ounce of spermicide is equal to six teaspoons or three applications. A 3.8-ounce tube contains about 11 applications. Make certain the contents are actually a spermicide. Some vaginal lubricants, which do not contain spermicidal ingredients, are sold in similar packages.

Contraceptive creams and jellies are often available at reduced cost from Planned Parenthood and some other family planning clinics.

If you need to replace your diaphragm, it's not necessary to have another pelvic examination, unless more than 12 months have passed since your last one. If you make a note of the size of your diaphragm, the health care practitioner who provided it can telephone a prescription for a new one to your pharmacy. The size is usually printed on the rim.

4

The Cervical Cap

The cervical cap is a small, deep rubber cup with a firm but flexible rim around the open end. It is 1¼ to 1½ inches long and looks like a large rubber thimble. It fits closely over the cervix and the os, the cervical opening.

Although the cervical cap functions like a diaphragm, it has a different shape, fits differently, and is used with less spermicide or none at all. It is held in place by suction, by its close fit on the cervix, and by the slight pressure of the surrounding vaginal wall. It has an important advantage over the diaphragm—you can insert the cap many hours before intercourse and leave it in place for a longer period of time afterward, although this practice may cause an odor. However, the only cap available currently in the United States— the Prentif cap—is made in only four sizes. Because anatomy varies, about 20 percent of women cannot get a good fit with this type of cap.

The cervical cap has been in use in Europe since the nineteenth century, but it was not approved by the FDA for general use in the United States until 1988. For this reason, many physicians are still unfamiliar with this method. Cervical caps are more likely to be available from women's health clinics.

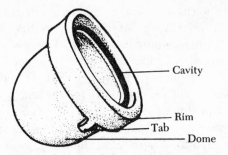

Figure 4.1 The Prentif Cervical Cap

EFFECTIVENESS

In studies of cap efficacy, failure rates range from 8 to 19 pregnancies per 100 women during the first year of use. As with other barrier contraceptives, the effectiveness of the cap depends largely on how faithfully it is used. To protect against pregnancy and disease, you must wear the cap for every act of intercourse outside of menstruation. (Use another method, such as a condom, at that time.)

A disadvantage of the cap is that it can become dislodged during intercourse if it hasn't been put on correctly in the first place or if it doesn't fit securely enough because of the shape of the cervix. You can sometimes avoid dislodgement by taking a different position during intercourse.

You can improve the effectiveness of the cervical cap by utilizing a backup method of contraception during the first few months of use. Your partner might use a condom on your most fertile days (see Chapter 13).

HEALTH EFFECTS

The cervical cap seldom causes negative health effects. There is a theoretical risk of toxic shock syndrome if you wear the cap for more than 72 hours, although no documented cases exist. Nevertheless, if you have a history of toxic shock syndrome, you should not use the cap. To avoid the possibility of toxic shock, do not wear the cap for more than 48 hours and do not use it during menstruation. Symptoms of toxic shock include fever, diarrhea, vomiting, muscle aches, and a sunburnlike rash that also involves the palms of the hands and the soles of the feet. If these occur, remove the cap immediately and notify your doctor.

In a study of cervical cap use sponsored by the National Institutes of Health, 4 percent of the women who entered the study with normal Pap tests developed cervical tissue abnormalities during their first three months of using the cap. Researchers theorize that the epithelium, the cell layer that lines the cervix, may become more vulnerable to the human papilloma virus with regular cervical cap use. (Several strains of human papilloma virus can lead to cancer of the cervix.) As a result, the FDA currently requires that a Pap test be per-

NOT EVERY WOMAN CAN WEAR A CERVICAL CAP

The Prentif is the only cap available on the market in the United States, and not all women can use it successfully. Prentif caps come in four sizes and do not fit all women, largely because of ordinary variations in the anatomy of the individual cervix.

If the cervix has uneven sides, is exceptionally long or short, or is irregularly shaped, it is usually impossible to achieve the snug fit that is necessary for effective birth control. If the uterus is anteflexed—bent so the cervix points back toward the spine—the cap could easily be dislodged.

Last, a woman may not be able to use a cervical cap because she has a very long vagina and cannot reach her cervix in order to place a cap on it. When the Dumas cap becomes available in the United States (probably in several years), it will be possible to fit more women with this type of barrier contraceptive.

formed before a cap is fitted and again after three months of use. If either test shows any abnormal cells, the cap should not be used.

There is always a slight risk that the cap may irritate the cervix. If you are allergic to a spermicide, switch to a different, unperfumed product or a product with a lower percentage of nonoxynol-9. If this approach is not successful, the next step is to switch to Koromex Cream, in which the active ingredient is octoxynol. (Unfortunately, octoxynol is similar to nonoxynol, so this change may not solve the problem.) If the irritation continues, the cause may be an allergy to the rubber in the cap. Any allergic reaction that appears to be caused by the cap or spermicide should be discussed with a doctor.

HOW TO USE THE CERVICAL CAP
Being Fitted

The Prentif is a deep cap, almost 1½ inches long. It is made of soft, natural rubber with a sturdy rim. Cut into the inside of the rim is a groove that enhances the cap's ability to cling to the cervix. The Prentif comes in four sizes: 22, 25, 28, and 31 millimeters in internal diameter.

The Dumas cap is shallower and thicker and is held in place by the walls of the vagina, somewhat like a small diaphragm. Made in diameters that range from 50 to 75 millimeters, it fits many women whose anatomy prevents them from wearing a Prentif cap. If your cervix is short or irregular in shape, or has uneven sides or considerable scarring, you may get a good fit with a Dumas cap, if you can find one in this country.

The best time to be fitted is the middle of the menstrual cycle, between days 10 and 18. (Day one is the first day of menstruation.) First, your health care provider will take your medical history, do a thorough pelvic examination, and perform a Pap test. The purpose is to discover any medical or anatomical problem involving the cervix, such as an inflamed or irregularly shaped cervix, that might lead to a serious infection or make it impossible for the cap to achieve a good seal. If you have had a pelvic exam and a Pap test within the preceding three months, just get a note or a copy of the test results from the practitioner who performed the exam.

Note: No matter what type of contraception you are using, you should have a Pap smear every year. This test can detect precancerous cervical changes and may also detect STDs and vaginal infections.

A cap cannot be fitted during pregnancy, during menstruation, or when a vaginal or cervical infection or inflammation is present. Nor can it be fitted during the weeks immediately following a birth or abortion or any procedure that involves the cervix, such as a dilation and curettage (D&C).

Because differences in anatomy affect the way the cap fits, it is a good idea to ask your practitioner just how well the cap covers your cervix. If the fit involves any idiosyncracies, you should be aware of them so you know when your cap is in the right place. For instance, if you have a long cervix, a cap might not completely cover it. If you have any question about cap placement or the security of its seal, if you are not sure you are inserting it correctly, or if it's uncomfortable, arrange for a fitting check after you have practiced with it at home.

To achieve a good fit, the inner diameter of the cap must be only a millimeter or two larger than the cervix. When the cap is on the cervix, there should be no space between the rim and the cervix, and the cap should be deep enough so its top does not rest on the os.

Using the Cap

Some women find inserting and removing a cervical cap a bit more difficult than using a diaphragm. Other women find that the cap requires less effort because it's smaller and easier to move through the vagina. With practice at home, most women are able to slide it into place quickly and easily. Take all the time you need at your doctor's office or clinic until you feel sure that you are putting the cap in and taking it out correctly. In addition, sitting in on a cervical cap self-help group—if one is available—helps to ensure receiving an adequate fit and being satisfied with this contraceptive method. Practitioners who fit caps are good sources for locating such groups.

To make sure it's comfortable, practice inserting the cap several times and wear it for eight hours before you actually use it for intercourse.

To test its fit, remove the cap after 20 minutes of wear and see if you can feel a raised ring around your cervix. If you can, the cap has a good, snug fit. If there's no ring, the cap may be too loose. If this occurs more than once, tell your clinician.

The Insertion Procedure. Before inserting your cap, empty your bladder and wash your hands. Choose a comfortable position: squatting; lying down with your legs bent; sitting on the edge of a sturdy chair; standing with one foot propped on a chair, the edge of the bathtub, or the toilet seat; sitting on the toilet. Experiment until you find the position that works best for you.

Fill one-third of the dome with spermicidal cream or jelly. Sometimes the cream may become rancid if the cap is left in for more than 48 hours; jelly doesn't. Fill the cap no more than one-third full; too much jelly or cream can prevent a good seal and may make it easier for the cap to come off during intercourse. Don't put spermicide into the hollow groove on the inside of the rim, but do put a dab of it in one spot on the outer rim to make it easier to slide into and up the vagina. You improve your protection if you add an applicator of spermicide to your vagina after you insert the cap.

Like the condom and the diaphragm, the cervical cap is rubber and so can be damaged by any oil-based substance. If you want to use a lubricant during intercourse, try K-Y Jelly, H-R Lubricating Jelly, Surgilube, or another water-based product, available in drugstores.

Before inserting the cap, locate your cervix with your fingers. Because its position changes throughout your menstrual cycle, knowing its current position makes it easier to put the cap in place.

Pinch the edges of the cap together between your thumb

and first finger. With your other hand spread apart the vaginal lips. Push the cap gently up into the vagina and along its back wall, with the opening facing up and the dome down. When your thumb can no longer reach far enough, use one or two of your longest fingers to move the cap along to the cervix. Push the cap on over the end of the cervix. Although this can be done with one finger, it's easier if you place the index finger on one side of the cap and the middle finger on the other side and push it on. Then use those fingers to press around the entire rim to make certain the cap is pushed as far as it will go and is securely in place.

If it's hard for you to reach your cervix, try squatting or bear down with your abdominal muscles as if you were having a bowel movement. This pressure pushes your cervix down lower into the vaginal canal. If you continue to have difficulty inserting the cap, remove it, relax, and try again. You may want to try another position. If you feel secure and comfortable before you begin, it's easier to insert the cap.

Checking the Placement. When the cap is in place, use your fingers as described above to make sure the cap is positioned

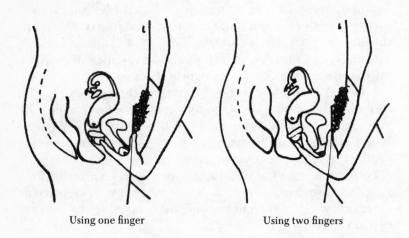

Using one finger   Using two fingers

Figure 4.2 Placing Cap on Cervix

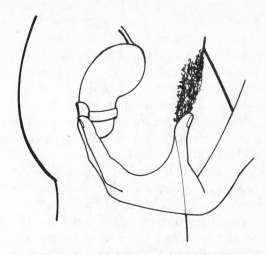

Figure 4.3 Checking Cap Placement

completely over the cervix. Experienced fitters recommend checking at the back of the cap, where the cervix is easier to feel and recognize. If the cap is on properly, it should completely cover the cervix up to the point where the cervix meets the vaginal walls. The cap shouldn't touch the tip of the cervix at all. The dome should not feel taut but should "dimple in" when touched. In order to find the cervix itself, you should have to reach a bit inside the rim of the cap, but you should not be able to knock the cap loose. A well-fitted cap is difficult to remove.

If the cap is not correctly positioned, either straighten it with your fingers or remove and reinsert it. Checking its position on the cervix is important because a cap can stick to the vaginal wall instead of sliding up to and on the cervix. Positioning the cap sounds much more difficult and complex than it actually is. With practice it soon becomes a quick, almost automatic act.

If the Cap Becomes Dislodged. Displacement of the cap occurs most often when the penis is able to reach the cervix. The angle of the cervix or the angle of penetration may cause the penis to bump the side of the cap rather than the dome, pushing it out of place. Soon after intercourse, check to see whether the cap is still in place. If it's loose, push it back on the cervix and immediately add an applicator of spermicide well back into the vagina. If it is completely dislodged, remove it, put some spermicide in the cap if necessary, and replace it. Then add the extra spermicide. If the cap becomes dislodged frequently, regardless of the positions you are using, see your practitioner. You may have to consider using another contraceptive method.

To put spermicide in the vagina, remove the top of the tube and attach the applicator in its place. Squeeze the tube until the applicator is full, disconnect it, and insert the applicator of spermicide well into your vaginal canal, just like a tampon. Gently push the plunger as far as it can go. Remove the applicator without tugging on the plunger, which can pull up some of the spermicide.

Insert the cap at least 20 to 30 minutes before intercourse so that a good seal can develop. If you've been wearing the cap for several hours before you have intercourse, make sure it is securely in place before you begin lovemaking. You can do this in bed, and either you or your partner can check its position.

Afterward. After intercourse, leave the cap in place for at least eight hours. If it's convenient, you can leave it in as long as a day or two. Most practitioners recommend that the cap not be worn more than two days at a time, largely because of the odor caused by vaginal secretions on the rubber. In addition, not enough is known about the long-term effects of blocking the flow of normal cervical secretions and the risk of toxic shock syndrome. However, some women can wear a cap almost constantly without a problem. They remove it every other day or once a day for a few hours to wash it and to allow cervical secretions to flow freely.

Do not douche while wearing a cervical cap, because you could dilute the spermicide or force sperm into the cap. The douching solution also might make holes in the rubber.

Wearing the Cap During Menstruation. It is not a good idea to wear the cap during those days of your period when blood flow is heavy. If blood spills over the rim, it breaks the seal between cap and cervix. Since it is remotely possible to become pregnant during menstruation, you or your partner should use another form of birth control at this time.

Further Intercourse. If you have intercourse again while the cap is still in place, add more spermicide.

For the first few weeks or months that you use the cap— until you feel certain you are using it correctly and know it will not become dislodged—back it up with spermicide or a condom. If the cap does become loose during intercourse, try different positions to find one that doesn't dislodge it. Use a backup contraceptive method while you are experimenting. If the cap still comes loose, return to your health care provider to try to resolve the problem.

Removing the Cap

To remove the cap, it's necessary to break the force of the seal. After you've been wearing the cap for some hours, the cervix swells slightly, creating an even tighter seal. With experience you will learn how much effort you need to loosen it.

After finding a comfortable position, hook a finger over the back rim of the cap and pull. Or push the dome of the cap forward with your index finger while your middle finger hooks over the back rim and pulls down. If you can't reach the cap, even when bearing down, ask your clinician for a prescription for the diaphragm introducer (the Universal Introducer). It has a small hook on one end that is useful for removing cervical caps.

Care and Storage

Wash the cap with a mild, unscented soap and warm water. Turn it inside out in order to clean the hollow groove in the rim. Use a strong flow of warm water or a soft toothbrush. *Do not boil the cap.* Dry the cap and, if you are not going to use it soon, dust it lightly with cornstarch to help protect the rubber from oily residues. *Do not use talcum or baby powders,* because they cause rubber to deteriorate. Scented powders also can irritate the walls of your vagina. Don't rest the cap on newsprint, because it may contain ingredients that can perforate rubber. Keep the cap away from extreme heat and sunlight because these too cause rubber to deteriorate. Store the cap in its container. If you accidentally drop the cap, simply wash it in soap and water.

If an unpleasant odor develops when you wear the cap for extended periods, you may need to remove it more often, perhaps at least once a day, for cleaning. You can often neutralize the odor by soaking the cap in lemon juice, mouthwash, or a mild solution of one teaspoon white or cider vinegar to a quart of water. Soak it for 20 minutes. The vinegar solution will turn the cap brown, but this darkening effect does not affect its reliability. Rinse the cap thoroughly in warm water and dry it. Odors also can be removed by adding a drop of liquid chlorophyll to the cap *before* using it or by soaking it in a cup of water mixed with a drop of chlorophyll. Chlorophyll is available from drugstores and some natural food stores. Do not soak a cap for more than 20 to 30 minutes.

If you have a vaginal infection, wash and sterilize the cap in rubbing alcohol for 15 minutes each time you remove it. It is also a good idea to have your partner wear a condom for his protection until the infection is cleared up.

The regular use of alcohol and acidic solutions, such as vinegar and water or lemon juice, hasten the deterioration of rubber caps. At the first sign of cracking, hardness, stickiness, or a persistent odor, get a new cap. Generally speaking, caps should be replaced every year. How long each one lasts depends on how often you use it, the effect of the body's secretions on the rubber, and how well you take care of it.

Checking the Cap. Every time you use your cap, examine it carefully for holes, cracks, and signs of wear. Hold it up to the light, or check for leaks by filling it with water. Also, have your cap checked at the time of your annual gynecological examination. Your health care provider may observe changes in the cap that you haven't noticed. The rubber may be subtly deteriorating, for example, or the shape may have altered so it is no longer providing a good seal.

The fit of a cap should also be tested after childbirth, a miscarriage, or an abortion. After a birth, the cervix takes about six weeks to return to its normal size. Furthermore, the fit of a cervical cap should be checked after any surgery on the cervix, including laser, electrocautery, or cryotherapy, and after any gynecological procedure in which the cervix has been dilated, such as a D&C. If you are breast-feeding when you are fitted with your cap, have the size checked when you are menstruating once again—your cervix may have become larger. And if you were fitted while you were on oral contraceptives, have the fit tested after you experience your first spontaneous period off the Pill.

Where to Get the Cervical Cap

Although more-populous states may have numerous health professionals trained to fit cervical caps, in other states the number of practitioners fitting caps is still relatively small, although the number continues to grow. For a provider near you, contact Cervical Cap Ltd., 430 Monterey Avenue, Los Gatos, CA 95030, 408-395-2100, for an updated list for your area.

Cost

A cervical cap itself ranges in cost from $30 to $40; the preliminary pelvic examination, Pap test, and fitting procedure will add another $50 to $100. Because using the cap requires much less spermicide, a tube of contraceptive cream or jelly is likely to last much longer than when used alone or with the diaphragm.

5

The Contraceptive Sponge

One of the most convenient barrier methods of birth control for a woman is the contraceptive sponge. The sponge is round, with a deep indentation on one side, and looks somewhat like a small, white doughnut. Made of a white polyurethane foam, the contraceptive sponge is placed high in the vagina over the cervix. It contains the spermicide nonoxynol-9, which slowly disperses over the cervix and upper vagina for up to 30 hours. The sponge is available in a single size: 2¼ inches in diameter and about ¾ inch thick. It fits most women who have never been pregnant. Unlike the diaphragm and cervical cap, the sponge does not require fitting by a doctor. Sponges are available in drugstores.

The presence of a spermicide and the fact that the sponge provides a barrier between the cervix and the penis do furnish a measure of protection against sexually transmitted diseases. The sponge contains a gram of nonoxynol-9. This is more than the amount contained in either an applicator of any spermicide, which holds an average of 150 milligrams (one thousandth of a gram), or in a spermicidal condom, which contains about 75 milligrams.

The sponge is inserted so it covers the os, somewhat like a diaphragm. It prevents pregnancy by killing the sperm with nonoxynol-9, by physically blocking sperm from the cervix, and by trapping sperm in the sponge. The most effective of these is the sponge's spermicidal action.

The large "dimple" in one side of the sponge fits over the cervix, which makes the sponge easier to fold for inserting. The spermicide is activated when the sponge is made wet; no extra spermicide or cream is needed, even for multiple acts of intercourse, and the sponge can be inserted many hours beforehand. After being left in place for at least six hours after the last intercourse, the sponge is gently pulled out of the vagina by its attached ribbon, much like a tampon. It can be used for only one 24-hour period, after which it is discarded. (It should not be flushed down the toilet.)

EFFECTIVENESS

According to several studies of the efficacy of the contraceptive sponge, the lowest first-year failure rate for the typical user varies from 14 percent for women who have never had a baby, to 28 percent for women who had given birth to at least one child. This rather high range of failures, however, included women who did not use the sponge for every act of intercourse and who may not have followed the directions exactly. The failures were fewest among women who used this method carefully and consistently, and who had never been pregnant.

The high incidence of failure for women who had given birth at least once may be due to the fact that pregnancy and a vaginal delivery stretch the vaginal canal and the cervix. A bigger vagina may allow the sponge to move out of place during intercourse, and the broader cervix may no longer be completely covered by the single-size sponge currently available. The failure rate for these women is notably high, so the sponge method is not recommended by many practitioners for women who have given birth. However, it is still better than no contraceptive at all. Effectiveness is further improved over the long term if you always use a second method during the most fertile days of your menstrual cycle.

Like other barrier methods, the sponge cannot protect against pregnancy if it is not used every time a woman has intercourse. On the other hand, because the sponge is inexpensive and does not interrupt lovemaking, some people may find it more attractive and use it more consistently.

HEALTH EFFECTS

Since the sponge contains a substantial amount of nonoxynol-9, a small percentage of women and men develop an allergic reaction—soreness or a reddish inflammation where their bodies have been in close contact with the spermicide. If this occurs, use a different contraceptive.

Although the chance of developing toxic shock syndrome while using a contraceptive sponge is extremely small, use another method of birth control, such as the condom, during your period or if you have any abnormal discharge or bleeding.

WHO SHOULDN'T USE THE SPONGE?

The contraceptive sponge should not be used after any pregnancy (whether or not it's been carried to full term) without a physical examination to determine if it provides effective protection. In general, the sponge is not recommended for women who have given birth. This is because of its high failure rate under these circumstances.

The sponge is not a good contraceptive for any woman who has had toxic shock syndrome. If either partner is allergic to nonoxynol-9, the sponge also is not recommended.

Because of its fairly substantial failure rate, the sponge is probably not a good contraceptive for a woman who absolutely does not want to get pregnant.

HOW TO USE A CONTRACEPTIVE SPONGE

The sponge is convenient because it can remain in the vagina for a total of 30 hours. Since it should be left in place for at least six hours after intercourse, this timing allows you to insert it any time up to 24 hours before you have sex. It is important not to wear the sponge for more than 30 hours, because the slight risk of toxic shock syndrome may be increased if secretions accumulate in the sponge and provide a focus for the infection.

Inserting the Sponge

Before removing the sponge from its airtight individual package, wash your hands. Then wet the sponge with about 2 tablespoons of clean tap water in order to activate the spermicide. Squeeze the sponge gently once or twice so it foams, *but do not squeeze it dry.* The sponge should feel sudsy but not drippy.

If you haven't used a contraceptive sponge before, you may want to practice inserting and removing one before you actually use it for birth control.

The way you position your body for receiving the contraceptive sponge is similar to that for inserting a diaphragm, cervical cap, or tampon. You can insert it while lying on your back with legs bent, sitting on the toilet, or squatting. (If this is your first use of a barrier contraceptive, refer to Figure 3.1, page 34, for instructions on how to insert a diaphragm.)

Hold the sponge in one hand with the indentation or "dimple" facing up and the removal loop dangling below. Pinch the sides together to make the sponge long and narrow. The loop should run underneath from front to back. Use your other hand to spread apart the vaginal lips. Then gently slide the folded sponge into the vagina and push it up with your middle finger until it reaches the cervix.

When you let go of it, the sponge will open out and fill the vagina. Push it up against the cervix so the sponge covers it

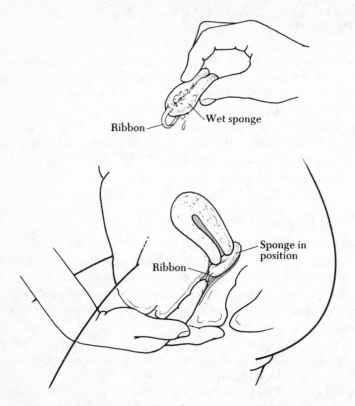

Figure 5.1 How to Insert the Contraceptive Sponge

all around. You should be able to feel the removal loop on the underside.

If the sponge doesn't appear to be covering the cervix, use your finger to move it around until no part of the cervix feels uncovered and the sponge reaches from side to side in the upper vagina. If you can't feel the loop underneath, it's best to remove the sponge and start over.

The first few times you use the sponge, putting it in place may take a few minutes. It is easier to insert than the diaphragm or cervical cap, and it's also less messy because you don't apply a spermicide yourself.

If the Sponge Becomes Dislodged

The muscles of the vagina hold the sponge firmly in place so it seldom becomes dislodged. As with a tampon, it is possible to swim and exercise vigorously while wearing it. Sometimes strong internal pushing, such as during a bowel movement, may cause it to slide down to the opening of the vagina. This is more likely to happen after intercourse, when the sponge is slippery with semen. If this happens, push it back up over the cervix with a finger. If it slips out of the vagina after intercourse, moisten a new sponge and insert it immediately.

Do not douche while the sponge is in the vagina. The douching solution will dilute the spermicide.

Further Intercourse

You can have intercourse as often as you like during the 24-hour period after inserting the sponge, and you don't have to add spermicide. After the last act of intercourse, don't remove the sponge for six hours.

If you anticipate further lovemaking after 24 hours have elapsed and six hours have passed since your last intercourse, remove the sponge and replace it with a new one.

Removing the Sponge

Before removing the sponge, wash your hands. Reach up into the vagina with a finger and find the removal loop. If you can't reach the loop, take a deep breath and bear down with your abdominal muscles to press your cervix closer to the vaginal opening so you can get a better grasp of the loop.

Hook your finger into the loop and slowly and gently pull the sponge down. (Don't jerk on the loop or the sponge.) If your vagina seems to be holding it tightly, stop, relax, and wait a moment or two before trying again. If the sponge still doesn't move, tighten your vaginal muscles as hard as you can while taking a deep breath. Keep the muscles clenched and hold your breath while you count to 10. Then *slowly* relax and breathe out. Repeat this once or twice. Then, as you breathe out and feel relaxed, bear down. Continue to relax your body as you reach in and remove the sponge. This technique works right away for some women; for others, it takes practice.

The sponge sometimes becomes so tightly fitted against the cervix that it takes a bit of effort to break the suction. Slip a fingertip between the *side edge* of the sponge and the vaginal wall, then break the suction by pulling the sponge away from the cervix. Bear down with your abdominal muscles so your finger can get better leverage on the sponge.

If the sponge was pushed to one side or turned during intercourse, the removal loop may be hard to find. Run your finger around the edge of the sponge until you discover the loop. Get your fingertip under the loop and slowly pull down on it. If you can't find the loop, bear down with your abdominal muscles so you can reach the sponge with two fingers, put one on either side, and gently pry it loose. Don't pull on the sponge itself, because it may tear.

What to Do If the Sponge Comes Apart

After you've removed the sponge, check to see whether it was torn during the removal process, particularly if it didn't come out easily. If it's torn or a piece is missing, use a finger to feel all around your vagina, particularly up around the cervix, to find the missing piece or pieces. Start near the cervix and sweep around all sides of the vagina, moving your finger gradually down toward the opening, and remove any bit of sponge you may feel. If you can't remove the sponge or its pieces, you may have to have them removed by a doctor.

The only sponge sold in the United States at the time of this writing is manufactured under the name Today. The manufacturer has a hotline telephone number (800-223-2329) and a trained staff to answer questions about the device and give guidance about inserting and removing it.

Cost

The Today sponge is sold in packages of three, six, and 12. Although prices vary from store to store, the approximate prices are $5, $9, and $15, respectively.

6

Spermicides

As the name implies, a spermicide is a chemical compound that kills sperm. Spermicides are available in a number of forms that are safe and easy to use—aerosol foams, creams, jellies, dissolvable suppositories, and dissolvable squares of film. The active ingredient in all but one of these products is nonoxynol-9. One cream, Koromex, is made for use with a diaphragm and contains octoxynol, a compound very similar to nonoxynol-9. Both chemicals work by fatally damaging the surface membrane of the sperm cell.

Like the contraceptive sponge, spermicides require no physical examination or prescription. They can be found in the feminine hygiene sections of drugstores, department stores, and many large supermarkets. They are also distributed by family planning clinics and some health care providers.

Although spermicides are effective when used alone, they offer more protection against sperm and disease when combined with another contraceptive, such as a condom or diaphragm. Like other barrier contraceptives, spermicides do not affect hormone levels in the body or change the environment of the uterus.

Vaginal spermicides are particularly useful as a temporary or backup method of birth control when other methods are not available. They can also provide protection when birth control pills are forgotten several days in a row or when the prescription hasn't been refilled in time. They are a good backup during the first weeks of using a condom, diaphragm, or cervical cap, while the man or woman becomes accustomed to using a new birth control method. And, at any time, if one method develops a problem, such as a condom tearing or a cervical cap becoming dislodged, an immediate application of spermicide may prevent conception.

EFFECTIVENESS

For typical users, spermicides have a first-year failure rate of 21 to 22 percent. Typical users include women who don't use the spermicide every time they have intercourse and women who don't always use it correctly.

Most spermicide failures are experienced by women who are at their peak reproductive years or have intercourse frequently. Fewest failures are encountered by women whose risk of pregnancy is reduced because they have intercourse less often or are over age 35 and are less fertile. At all ages, conscientious use of a spermicide improves its effectiveness.

HEALTH EFFECTS

Some users find that a spermicide can irritate the vagina or the penis. Others may have an allergic reaction to the active agent or to the perfumes in a particular product. Symptoms can range from redness and itching to ulcerations that bleed. An allergy or irritation sometimes can be resolved by trying another brand or type of spermicide, one that has a different fragrance or none at all, or a product that uses octoxynol instead of nonoxynol-9. If these efforts do not help, stop using the product and discuss the problem with your health care provider. You may need to switch to a birth control method that does not include a spermicide.

WHO SHOULD NOT DEPEND ON SPERMICIDES?

Spermicides should not be used as the sole method of contraception by a woman who absolutely does not want to become pregnant. If you *must* avoid pregnancy for medical reasons, discuss with your physician which contraceptive method or combination of methods is best for you.

A thorough review of all available data has led medical experts to conclude that the use of spermicides does not affect subsequent pregnancies. Previous reports of spontaneous abortions and children born with birth defects among women using spermicides have not held up in recent studies.

SPERMICIDES AND HOW TO USE THEM

Creams, Jellies, and Foams

A variety of jellies, creams, and foams are available. Starter packages contain spermicide plus reusable applicators; refill packages do not include applicators. Conceptrol Gel Disposables offer individual applicators prefilled with contraceptive jelly for one-time use.

Some products are made to be used primarily with the additional protection of a diaphragm or condom. Other jellies are formulated to be used alone, and an applicator of these generally contains more nonoxynol-9 than an applicator of a jelly designed to accompany a diaphragm or condom. Read the label carefully to be sure you're getting what you want.

Normal body temperature melts these spermicides, allowing them to spread around the vagina and over the opening to the cervix. Melting takes place within minutes, so spermicides are effective almost immediately after application. For full protection, apply the spermicide high in the vagina, close to the cervix.

For creams and jellies, remove the screw-on top of the tube, twisting on the applicator in its place. Squeeze the tube to fill the applicator until the plunger is pushed out completely. Then gently insert the applicator deep into the vagina and push in the plunger as far as it will go. Remove the applicator by its barrel. Pulling on the plunger may cause it to suction out some of the spermicide.

Creams and jellies are effective for one hour. If more than an hour passes before intercourse, insert another applicator of spermicide. Each additional act of intercourse calls for more spermicide. Do not douche for at least six hours after intercourse. A tampon or minipad used after lovemaking protects against any leakage.

Contraceptive foams are available in pressurized aerosol cans. Before using, shake the can to mix the spermicide through the foam (the spermicide tends to settle in the bottom of the can). The foam should have the consistency of shaving cream—the more bubbles it has, the better it blocks sperm.

To fill the plunger-type plastic applicator, place it on the can of foam and either push or tilt it so foam flows into it. As the applicator fills, the foam pushes up the plunger. (The filling technique varies from brand to brand, and each package has directions explaining how to use it.) When full, insert the applicator deep into the vagina and push the plunger in until it stops. Remove the applicator with the plunger still pushed in to avoid withdrawing any of the foam.

The amount of active ingredient varies from product to product. It is important to use the applicator that comes with a particular spermicide, because the applicator provides the correct dose for its product only. Application may differ from product to product.

Care and Storage. Wash the applicator thoroughly inside and out with hot water and soap or detergent. Do not boil because it is plastic and likely to melt. To keep it clean, store in the original box or in a tightly closed plastic bag. Store all spermicides at room temperature, away from extreme heat or cold. They should not be used more than two years after purchase or beyond the expiration date marked on the package.

With some brands of foam it's impossible to know how much remains in the can after a few applications. Certain brands provide a mechanism for checking to see how much spermicide is left. To make sure you don't run out of foam, first buy two containers and then buy another as soon as one becomes empty.

Cost. Creams and jellies range in cost from $7 to $13, depending on size. Foams cost between $9 and $11 per can. In general, refill tubes sold without applicators offer the most spermicide for the money.

Vaginal Suppositories

Vaginal suppositories resemble large pills. They are pushed with a finger well up into the vagina, where they melt or foam, allowing the nonoxynol-9 to spread around the upper vagina and over the opening of the cervix. Depending on the brand, they must be inserted 10 or 15 minutes before intercourse takes place and are effective for one hour. You must insert a new tablet for every additional act of intercourse and whenever intercourse is delayed beyond the one-hour limit. As noted above, do not douche for at least six hours after your partner's last ejaculation. Suppositories dissolve completely in the vagina, and leakage seldom is a problem.

The Encare suppository does not melt but instead foams as it dissolves. In some women, this foaming action creates an uncomfortable feeling of warmth in the vagina.

Keep suppositories away from extreme cold or heat and store at room temperature. If a tablet melts, leave it in its plastic casing in a cool place, such as the refrigerator, for about an hour, and it will regain its shape and firmness.

Suppositories cost about 60 to 75 cents apiece and are sold in packages of 10, 12, and 20 tablets. They are the least

AVA

VAGINAL SPERMICIDES AVAILABLE

Product	Manufacturer	Active Ingredient	Concentration (percentage)
Creams			
Koromex Cream*	Schmid	Octoxynol	3
Ortho-Creme*	Ortho	Nonoxynol-9	2
Jellies			
Conceptrol Gel Disposables	Ortho	Nonoxynol-9	4
Gynol II Extra Strength	Ortho	Nonoxynol-9	3
Gynol II Original Formula*	Ortho	Nonoxynol-9	2
Gynol II Starter*	Ortho	Nonoxynol-9	2
Ortho-Gynol*	Ortho	Nonoxynol-9	1
Koromex Crystal Clear Gel*	Schmid	Nonoxynol-9	3
Koromex Jelly	Schmid	Nonoxynol-9	3
Ramses Crystal Clear Gel	Schmid	Nonoxynol-9	5
Foams (used without diaphragm)			
Delfen Contraceptive Foam	Ortho	Nonoxynol-9	12.5
Emko Because	Schering	Nonoxynol-9	8
Emko Vaginal Contraceptive Foam	Schering	Nonoxynol-9	8
Koromex Foam	Schmid	Nonoxynol-9	12.5
Vaginal Inserts			
Encare	Thompson	Nonoxynol-9	2.27
Koromex Vaginal Inserts	Schmid	Nonoxynol-9	5
Semicid	Whitehall	Nonoxynol-9	6.25
Contraceptive Film			
Vaginal Contraceptive Film	Apothecus	Nonoxynol-9	28

*To be used with a diaphragm or condom; not to be used alone.

expensive of all the forms of spermicides, and the packages are small enough to carry in a pocket or purse.

Contraceptive Film

Vaginal contraceptive film is one of the newest spermicidal products available. Each film is 2 inches square, very thin, and flexible. Like a vaginal suppository, it is pushed up as close to the cervix as possible. Body warmth melts the film, transforming it into a sperm-killing jelly within 15 minutes. It is then effective for up to two hours. Another film must be used if intercourse is desired after that time. After a few more hours, the jelly is completely dissolved by vaginal secretions, and leakage seldom is a problem.

Contraceptive film is sold in a compact box of 12 that is not much larger than a matchbook. The cost is about $8 per box.

Two

▲▽▲

Hormonal Methods

7

The Pill: Combined Oral Contraceptives

Birth control pills, also called oral contraceptives, offer almost complete protection against pregnancy when taken as prescribed. They are available in several types and in more than 30 different formulations. Most common are the "combination" pills, which contain synthetic versions of the two major types of female hormones: estrogens and progestins. Combination pills come in three models: single phase, biphasic, and triphasic. All contain an estrogen and a progestin, but the biphasic and triphasic pills provide the hormones in amounts that vary from one phase of the monthly cycle to another, in an effort to mimic a woman's natural hormonal cycle. In addition to the combination pill, there is the minipill, which contains only a progestin (see Chapter 8).

Birth control pills can be prescribed by physicians, nursemidwives, nurse-practitioners, and physician's assistants working in public and private clinics and health care offices.

COMBINATION PILLS

As explained in the chapter on anatomy, the process of ovulation is directed by hormones, messenger chemicals made by the body. Monthly changes in the production of several hormones, which act in a highly synchronized sequence, cause an

AVA

AVAILABLE ORAL CONTRACEPTIVES

PHASIC ORAL CONTRACEPTIVES

Product		Progestin Dose (mg)[a]	Estrogen Dose (mcg)[b]	Manufacturer
Ortho-Novum 7/7/7	First 7 days	0.5	35	Ortho
21- and 28-day packs	Next 7 days	0.75	35	
	Next 7 days	1	35	
Ortho-Novum 10/11	First 10 days	0.5	35	Ortho
21- and 28-day packs	Next 11 days	1	35	
Tri-Levlen	First 6 days	0.05	30	Berlex
21- and 28-day packs	Next 5 days	0.075	40	
	Next 10 days	0.125	30	
Tri-Norinyl	First 7 days	0.5	35	Syntex
21- and 28-day packs	Next 9 days	1.0	35	
	Next 5 days	0.5	35	
Triphasil	First 6 days	0.05	30	Wyeth-Ayerst
21- and 28-day packs	Next 5 days	0.075	40	
	Next 10 days	0.125	30	

CONSTANT-DOSE ORAL CONTRACEPTIVES

Product	Progestin Dose (mg)[a]	Estrogen Dose (mcg)[b]	Manufacturer
Brevicon 21- and 28-day packs	0.5	35	Syntex
Demulen 1/35 21- and 28-day packs	1	35	Searle
Levlen 21- and 28-day packs	0.15	30	Berlex
Loestrin 1/20 21- and 28-day packs	1	20	Parke-Davis
Loestrin 1.5/30 21- and 28-day packs	1.5	30	Parke-Davis
Lo/Ovral 21- and 28-day packs	0.3	30	Wyeth-Ayerst
Modicon 21- and 28-day packs	0.5	35	Ortho
Nordette 21- and 28-day packs	0.15	30	Wyeth-Ayerst
Norethin 1/35 21- and 28-day packs	1	35	Schiapparelli Searle
Norinyl 1+35 21- and 28-day packs	1	35	Syntex

△▽

AVAILABLE ORAL CONTRACEPTIVES

PHASIC ORAL CONTRACEPTIVES

Product	Progestin Dose (mg)[a]	Estrogen Dose (mcg)[b]	Manufacturer
Ortho-Novum 1/35 21- and 28-day packs	1	35	Ortho
Ovcon 35 21- and 28-day packs	0.4	35	Mead Johnson

ORAL CONTRACEPTIVES WITH 50 MCG OF ESTROGEN

	Progestin Dose (mg)[a]	Estrogen Dose (mcg)[b]	Manufacturer
Demulen 21- and 28-day packs	1	50	Searle
Norethin 1/50 21- and 28-day packs	1	50	Schiapparelli Searle
Norinyl 1+50 21- and 28-day packs	1	50	Syntex
Norlestrin 1/50 21- and 28-day packs	1	50	Parke-Davis
Norlestrin 2.5/50 21-day pack	2.5	50	Parke-Davis
Ortho-Novum 1/50 21- and 28-day packs	1	50	Ortho
Ovcon 50 21- and 28-day packs	1	50	Mead Johnson
Ovral 21- and 28-day packs	0.5	50	Wyeth-Ayerst

[a]mg = milligram or 1 thousandth of a gram
[b]mcg = microgram or 1 millionth of a gram
Some oral contraceptives contain an iron supplement.

egg to mature in one of the ovaries and then to be released (ovulated). Other cyclical alterations in hormones cause the lining of the uterus to thicken with blood-rich tissue every month, in preparation for nurturing a fertilized egg.

All combination pills contain synthetic estrogen and progestin. They are taken for three consecutive weeks; during the fourth week either no pills or blank pills are taken, causing withdrawal bleeding, which is like a light menstruation. The Pill prevents pregnancy through several different mechanisms but chiefly by suppressing ovulation because of the intake of estrogen. Without an egg, pregnancy cannot take place.

In addition, the progestin in the Pill causes the cervical mucus to remain thick and sticky all month, making it very difficult for sperm to get through the cervix to the uterus.

The combination pill is one of the most effective reversible methods of birth control available today in the United States. There are definite advantages to pills with both hormones. The estrogen helps to stabilize the lining of the uterus—the endometrium—so that it is less likely to shed between menstrual cycles and cause breakthrough bleeding. The progestin is important to balance the estrogen that is being produced naturally by the body and supplied by the Pill. These hormones provide some of the important health benefits described later in this chapter.

Over the years, changes have been made in the amounts of estrogen and progestin contained in the Pill, as well as in the dosing schedules. Almost all oral contraceptives now contain markedly reduced levels of both hormones. Furthermore, the phasic oral contraceptives deliver the hormones in reduced amounts that more closely resemble natural, day-to-day hormone levels. Although triphasic pills are becoming popular, the older, single-phase (constant-dose) pills are still prescribed most often.

The Biphasic Pill

The first phased oral contraceptive, Ortho-Novum 10/11, was biphasic. This means the pills taken for the first 10 days of the month contain 0.5 milligram (mg, one thousandth of a gram) of progestin, and the last 11 pills in the cycle contain 1.0 milligram. The estrogen dose remains steady throughout the cycle at 35 micrograms (mcg, one millionth of a gram). The successful introduction of the biphasic pill some years ago led to the development of triphasic pills. Biphasics are still available, though.

The Triphasic Pill

In the triphasic (three-phase) pill, the amounts of estrogen and progestin change during the month. Phasic pills are promoted as mimicking a woman's natural hormone cycle, although the various brands take different approaches to doing so. One product, Ortho-Novum 7/7/7, for instance, uses the same amount of estrogen, 35 mcg, throughout the month. The amount of the progestin changes every seven days: the first seven pills contain 0.5 mg, the next seven contain 0.75 mg, and the last seven have 1 mg. Two other brands, Triphasil and Tri-Levlen, use a somewhat more potent synthetic progestin, in doses of 0.05 mg for the first six days, 0.075 mg for the next five days, and 0.125 mg for the last 10 days. The dose of estrogen in these brands also changes from phase to phase: from 30 mcg to 40 mcg to 30 mcg. Each phase is indicated by pill color. The amount of hormone and the phase lengths of another brand, Tri-Norinyl, are different still.

The dosage and scheduling differences among the pills have led some experts to question the validity of such cycling. If the manufacturers of oral contraceptives were truly trying to copy a woman's natural cycle, these critics point out, the triphasics would all follow a similar pattern. Moreover, regardless of their daily dosage levels, the phasic and older single-phase pills function the same way: They prevent ovulation and alter the cervical mucus and endometrium. The total amount of estrogen and progestin that phasic pills provide over the course of a month is only a little less than the hormones in a month's supply of any low-dose combination pill. At this time there appears to be little difference in efficacy and safety between the new phasic oral contraceptives and the traditional combination pills.

Triphasic pills have one drawback: The three phases of different-colored pills sometimes can be difficult to figure out, especially for women who are new to oral contraceptives.

HOW EFFECTIVE IS THE PILL?

When taken every day at approximately the same time, an oral contraceptive that includes synthetic estrogen is extremely effective. A pill that contains at least 30 mcg of estrogen has about a 1 to 2 percent failure rate. Pills containing 20 mcg of estrogen have a failure rate of 2 percent.

Among typical users, who may forget a pill occasionally, oral contraception is slightly less effective. Data on typical users of a combination pill reveal a failure rate of 3 percent during the first year of use. Women under age 22 have a slightly higher failure rate, 4.7 percent. (For protection against sexually transmitted diseases, pill users also need a barrier contraceptive.)

HOW REVERSIBLE IS THE PILL?

Generally speaking, if you are fertile before you begin using the Pill, your ability to conceive is not affected. Many women become pregnant within several months of stopping the Pill; for a substantial proportion of women, conception may take six months to a year and sometimes longer. The length of time the birth control pills have been used does not appear to affect how long it takes a woman to return to fertility.

Some women discover after discontinuing oral contraception that their periods do not return for several months. Any inability to conceive appears not to be related to the Pill itself but to the woman's age or other physical conditions that may have developed during Pill use.

RISKS AND BENEFITS
Possible Risks of the Pill

Virtually all the research on long-term complications of the Pill is based on the earlier combination pills that contained high doses of estrogen and progestin. Whether the new low-dose pills have the same complications and benefits will not be known until long-term studies of their effects are undertaken.

A few short-term and laboratory studies of the newer oral contraceptives suggest, however, that cardiovascular risks have declined as estrogen and progestin levels in the Pill have decreased. Furthermore, fewer women on low-dose pills complain about side effects such as breast swelling, nausea, and changes in skin pigmentation.

Anyone taking the Pill should be aware of the possible complications associated with its use and related symptoms. Pill users should discuss with their health care providers any physical or emotional changes that may be associated with Pill use.

Cardiovascular Disease. The estrogen in the Pill can foster the formation of blood clots, increasing their presence in the blood vessels. The changes in blood lipids that progestins can cause are associated with the development of fatty plaques in the inner lining of the arteries. The early high-dose oral contraceptives produced a slight but definite increase in the incidence of cardiovascular disorders. Moreover, the risk of death from these diseases was higher in women who also smoked and were over age 35. The present low-dose pills do not seem to cause any increase in cardiovascular disease among healthy nonsmoking women.

In the 1970s and early 1980s, there were occasional serious complications associated with the use of oral contraceptives: heart attack, pulmonary or cerebral embolism, and cerebral hemorrhage. A heart attack takes place when an area of heart muscle is deprived of blood, usually because a blood clot is blocking one of the coronary arteries. An embolism is a clump of material traveling in the bloodstream; blood clots are the most common. As the embolism moves through the blood vessels, it may become stuck and block the blood from reaching the parts of the body beyond it. A pulmonary embolism occurs when a blood clot is trapped in an artery going to the lungs, reducing their blood supply. When a cerebral embolism blocks one of the arteries that supplies the brain with oxygen-carrying blood, it causes a stroke.

Since the relationship between the early birth control pills and diseases of the heart and blood vessels became known, the amounts of estrogen and progestin in the various pills have been lowered, and today pills with the lowest amount of these hormones dominate the market. Because of the danger of cardiovascular disease, however, *a woman who wants to use even low-dose pills should stop smoking, regardless of her age.* The risk of heart attack is increased nearly 12-fold in women who smoke. When women smoke and take the Pill, the risk of a heart attack increases 50-fold.

Regardless of the type of oral contraceptive used, the chance of developing cardiovascular complications is increased for those who already have such health problems as high blood pressure, diseases of the heart or blood vessels, or poor circulation due to severe diabetes.

Breast Cancer. The connection between birth control pills and breast cancer has been the subject of more than 30 studies. Although a number of investigations found a somewhat elevated risk of breast cancer in some women who had at one time taken the Pill, the inconsistencies among results prevented researchers from concluding that the increased risks were definitely due to the Pill. The majority of the studies found no association at all between oral contraceptives and breast cancer. Five groups of experts reviewed the breast cancer/oral contraceptive data and found no clear-cut association between breast cancer and use of the Pill.

In January 1989 the FDA's Fertility and Maternal Health Drug Advisory Committee, one of the groups that reviewed the studies, stated that the link between breast cancer and certain long-term pill users found by several research groups was not a clear one and was inconsistent with other similar studies. The committee also pointed out that birth control pills provide many proven health benefits. It emphasized, however, that women who take oral contraceptives and also have a strong family history of breast cancer, small breast lumps, or abnormal mammograms should always be followed carefully by their physicians.

Cervical Dysplasia. Recent studies show that women who use oral contraceptives may be at a somewhat increased risk of cervical dysplasia (abnormal cell changes) and invasive cancer of the cervix. The dysplasia that precedes the development of cervical cancer can almost always be uncovered by an annual Pap test. Mild dysplasia may clear up on its own; more severe dysplasia and the early stages of actual cervical cancer can be treated and cured if detected promptly.

Chlamydial Cervicitis. Birth control pills can cause a condition called cervical erosion. The cervix is not actually eroded; instead, the cells that usually line the inside of the cervical canal migrate out and around the os, the mouth of the cervix. These cells are more vulnerable to chlamydial infections. There does not appear to be a corresponding increased risk of pelvic inflammatory disease, which is often associated with chlamydial infection, possibly because the progestin in the Pill thickens the cervical mucus so the chlamydial organisms are less able to get up into the genital tract and reach the fallopian tubes. Chlamydial cervicitis can be detected by a cervical swab.

Gallbladder Disease. The Pill may accelerate gallbladder problems for women who are prone to this disorder, so that gallstones become evident earlier. If you have a history of digestive disturbances or abdominal pain that suggests the presence of the disease, or have been diagnosed as actually having gallstones, you should not use any oral contraceptives containing estrogen, because this side effect appears to be estrogen-related.

High Blood Pressure. If you have experienced a rise in blood pressure during pregnancy, or have a strong family history of early hypertension, you should choose another contraceptive. If your current blood pressure is borderline high, you may not be a good candidate for oral contraceptives. But if you very much prefer using the Pill, have your blood pressure checked at regular intervals, and use a Pill that contains the lowest levels of hormones. You should also make every effort to reduce or eliminate life-style factors that may encourage hypertension: Lose weight if necessary, exercise regularly, reduce salt intake, cut down on caffeine, and reduce stress as much as possible.

Liver Tumors. The Pill has been associated with an increase in the incidence of very rare liver tumors that, even when benign, can lead to the rupture of the liver. The Pill also has been linked to rare occurrences of liver cancer. If you have liver disease or impaired liver function, do not take the Pill. The hormones are metabolized by the liver, which puts additional stress on that organ. But do use another method to protect yourself against conception, because pregnancy also stresses the liver.

Common Complaints or Side Effects

Some 40 percent of Pill users experience some side effects. Many of the minor ones subside after a few months. If they continue longer than three months, talk to your practitioner about switching to a different pill. *Continue taking the pills you have, however, until the prescription is changed or you start a new contraceptive.*

Nausea. Although nausea is not a common problem with the lower-dose pills, it does occur. Women experience it most often during their first month on the Pill or with the first few pills of each new package. It seldom is severe enough to cause vomiting. Many women find they can reduce nausea by taking the Pill at bedtime, with a meal, or with an evening snack. If nausea occurs for the first time after months or years of being on the Pill, it may be a sign of pregnancy.

Breast-feeding Problems. In nursing women, combined birth control pills diminish the quantity of breast milk. Furthermore, the hormones in the Pill pass into the milk in small amounts. Experts conclude that breast-feeding women should avoid using combination oral contraceptives if possible. But if you do use them, don't start until you have established a good flow of breast milk. Progestin-only oral contraceptives are a better choice for the nursing mother because they do not diminish the milk supply. (See Chapter 17 for more information on breast-feeding and contraceptive use.)

Headaches. While taking the Pill, some women develop severe, long-lasting, or recurrent headaches. Women who are prone to migraines may notice an increased severity in their headaches, although there is no solid evidence that the Pill increases the incidence of migraine. If headaches are severe and persistent, discuss them with your practitioner. It is possible you should use another form of contraception. If you have occasional migraines that are not too severe, a Pill with a lower estrogen content may resolve the problem.

Breast Swelling. Breast swelling is an effect of estrogen that women may experience naturally during their monthly cycle. Today's low-dose pills are much less likely to cause breast swelling. If it does occur, it can be a sign of pregnancy.

Fluid Retention. Oral contraceptives may cause you to retain fluid, resulting in swollen fingers and ankles. Bring these changes to the attention of your health care provider.

Weight Gain. The progestin in the Pill can cause an increase in appetite and consequent weight gain, but usually results only in an extra two to four pounds of added weight.

Depression. A large-scale British study in 1985 reported no difference in the incidence of depression among women who were on the Pill and women who used other forms of birth control. Women with a history of depression or psychiatric illness are more likely, however, to experience an exacerbation of their problem while using the Pill.

Interest in Sex. Conflicting reports exist about the effect of the birth control pill on sexual desire. Some Pill users say that their interest in sex diminishes. There are also anecdotal accounts that the premenstrual increase in libido experienced by some women disappears—that sexual urges flatten out instead of being cyclical during the month. Some women may have less lubrication in the vagina during lovemaking, which can make intercourse uncomfortable and even painful. Others enjoy sex more and have intercourse more often, probably because of a reduced fear of getting pregnant.

Contact Lens Problems. A contact lens wearer may experience changes in her vision or find she no longer is comfortable wearing her lenses. If these problems occur, she should consult her practitioner.

Skin Changes. Changes in the pigment of facial skin, in the form of a faint, brownish discoloration over the cheekbones, forehead, and upper lip, occur in some women taking oral contraceptives. These pigment changes are intensified by sunlight. Known as chloasma or melasma, this masklike marking fades in most cases in a few months to a few years. There is no treatment, but avoiding sunlight or using a strong sunblock may help.

Menstrual Disturbances

Scanty or Missed Periods. The monthly proliferation of blood and tissue in the lining of the uterus is almost always reduced in women who take birth control pills. The amount of blood lost during menstruation decreases accordingly. Very rarely, no bleeding occurs at all during the days the Pill is not taken. (This outcome is observed more often with the progestin-only pill.) If no bleeding occurs in your monthly cycle, it is important to contact your doctor—this may be a sign of pregnancy.

Breakthrough Bleeding or Spotting. When vaginal bleeding or staining occurs between periods, it is called breakthrough bleeding. This happens more often among women who are on very low-dose and progestin-only pills than among the users of standard combined oral contraceptives. It is more an annoyance than a medical problem. Most breakthrough bleeding occurs during the first months on the Pill. With low doses of estrogen, the endometrium becomes so thin it breaks loose from the uterus before menstruation is expected. With low-dose and progestin-only pills, breakthrough bleeding can be caused by missing a single pill or by not taking it at the same time every day. If you experience this problem, it is important to continue taking your pills on schedule. If the bleeding occurs in more than one cycle or lasts for more than a few days, talk to your practitioner.

Breakthrough bleeding also can appear after you have been on the Pill for a long time. If it occurs early in the cycle, some health care professionals may prescribe a small amount of extra estrogen to stop it. If it occurs later, they may suggest a pill with a stronger form of progestin, to give additional, late-cycle support to the endometrium.

Before your practitioner decides on treatment, you should have a physical examination to rule out other possible causes, such as a benign growth or a cancer. If the physical, including a Pap test, reveals no other possible reason for the bleeding, you could switch to a higher-dose pill, or you may be able to ignore the bleeding, if it is light and minor.

If breakthrough bleeding continues despite treatment, use another method of birth control and stop the Pill. If this approach does not eliminate the problem, more tests are called for in order to find the cause.

Early Menstruation. Another form of breakthrough bleeding is menstruation that begins a day or two before you stop taking the monthly schedule of active pills. Continue to take your pills on schedule. If this happens often, check with your practitioner, who may suggest that you take extra estrogen so the endometrium remains in place longer.

THE PILL'S PROTECTIVE EFFECTS

The Pill has protective effects against some common disorders:

- benign breast disease (fibrocystic disease)
- cancer of the ovaries
- cancer of the endometrium
- functional ovarian cysts
- iron deficiency anemia caused by heavy menstruation
- pelvic inflammatory disease
- pregnancy in the fallopian tubes (ectopic pregnancy)
- irregular menstrual cycles

Almost all the studies that demonstrated the protective effects of the Pill were done when most women were taking high-dose oral contraceptives. Although long-term studies of lower-dose formulations are not available, it is likely that a similar array of benefits—with fewer side effects—are associated with lower-dose pills.

Benign Breast Disease

Also known as *fibrocystic disease*, benign breast disease is the most common cause of a nonmalignant breast lump. The breast feels lumpy and may be tender in the days just before a menstrual period. Women who take birth control pills have fewer cases of fibrocystic disease. The incidence of this disorder is reduced the most for women who take pills that contain larger amounts of progestin. Protection increases with the number of years that oral contraceptives are used and persists for at least one year after they are discontinued.

Cancer of the Ovaries and Endometrium

The Pill also protects women against cancer of the ovaries and endometrial cancer of the uterus. Ovarian cancer is the fourth leading cause of cancer death in women and is particularly worrisome because it usually produces no symptoms until it is too late. It is fatal in almost 80 percent of the women who develop it. The incidence of ovarian cancer has been linked by some experts to *incessant ovulation,* an expression used to describe long stretches of ovulatory function uninterrupted by pregnancy and lactation. This is more common today than when women were frequently pregnant and breast-feeding—and thus not ovulating for a large percentage of their reproductive years. By stopping the ovulation process, it is theorized, birth control pills protect against ovarian cancer. The risk of ovarian cancer in women who have ever used the Pill is reduced by 40 percent.

Cancer of the endometrium is also common, occurring more often in women who, for a variety of reasons, have high blood levels of estrogen, often accompanied by low levels of progesterone and by incomplete sloughing of the uterine lining during bleeding. The use of oral contraceptives containing progestin lessens the risk of endometrial cancer, even when the Pill is used for only a short time. The risk of endometrial cancer in women who have ever used the Pill is reduced by 50 percent.

The protective effect of the combination pill against both endometrial and ovarian cancers increases with longer use. It is assumed that the positive effects of progestin-only pills also increase over time, although no studies document this belief.

Functional Ovarian Cysts

During the course of the menstrual cycle, some ovarian follicles respond to hormonal stimulation by continuing to grow instead of rupturing and releasing an egg or else simply disappearing at the end of the cycle. They are called functional cysts. "Functional" means the cyst is not pathological but is due to the function of the normal cycle. Many times there are no symptoms, but some cysts cause a variety of problems, including abdominal pain, pain during intercourse, and menstrual difficulties including delayed menstruation. In three epidemiological studies, the risk of functional ovarian cysts was reduced by the use of birth control pills, probably because of their effect in suppressing the hormonal events that stimulate ovulation. In a British study, the Pill led to a 64 percent drop in the incidence of these cysts.

Iron Deficiency Anemia

Iron is essential to the production of hemoglobin, the part of a red blood cell that transports oxygen from the lungs to the tissues, where the oxygen provides energy for vital chemical reactions in the cell. If dietary iron is insufficient or blood loss drains iron from the body, iron deficiency anemia can result. Mild iron deficiencies usually produce few or no symptoms, but moderate to severe iron deficiency anemia can cause lethargy and tiredness. More severe forms can cause dizziness, breathing difficulties during physical effort, and angina.

Oral contraceptives that combine estrogen and progestin inhibit the normal cyclical development of the lining of the uterus, in which the endometrium becomes enriched with extra blood in preparation for the implanting of an embryo. When this process does not occur, the amount of bleeding during menstruation is considerably diminished. Heavy periods, a frequent cause of iron deficiency anemia in women, are less common in Pill users. With the monthly blood loss reduced, the chance of becoming anemic is also decreased.

Pelvic Inflammatory Disease

Approximately one million women in the United States experience episodes of pelvic inflammatory disease (PID) every year; PID is an infection of the reproductive organs that often follows a sexually transmitted disease. Certain sexually transmitted diseases, such as chlamydia and gonorrhea (the most frequent causes of PID), have few or no symptoms in a woman's lower genital tract. If not treated, they can spread upward through the rest of the reproductive tract, involving the fallopian tubes and leaving scar tissue behind. Every bout of PID does additional damage, increasing a woman's chance of being infertile or having an ectopic pregnancy.

A major U.S. study of PID in users of oral contraceptives indicated that women who used the Pill had one-half the risk of PID, compared with women in their age group who did not use oral contraceptives. If a woman was on the Pill for at least one year, her risk was reduced by 70 percent. Although the actual mechanism for this protection is not known, researchers believe the thickening of the cervical mucus that occurs during Pill use probably inhibits infectious organisms from entering the upper reproductive system. Because the Pill can also reduce the length of the menstrual period and the amount of blood flow, it is theorized that these reductions may lessen the number of organisms using the blood as a growth medium when they are in the uterus. In addition, the inflammation and the scarring of the infection itself are reduced in Pill users.

It should be noted, however, that although the Pill may protect the upper reproductive system against the inflammation and scarring of the PID caused by sexually transmitted diseases, it offers no protection against lower genital infections by gonorrhea, chlamydia, syphilis, genital herpes, hepatitis B, and the AIDS virus.

Ectopic Pregnancy

When a pregnancy develops outside the uterus, usually in a fallopian tube, it is called an *ectopic*, or out-of-place, pregnancy. About one in every 100 pregnancies in the United States at this time is ectopic. The incidence is more common in women whose fallopian tubes are abnormal or are blocked by scar tissue. A fertilized egg may implant in a fallopian tube if a tubal abnormality prevents it from moving down into the uterus. Because the combination pill stops ovulation, it therefore protects against ectopic pregnancy.

Menstrual Cycle Benefits

The Pill provides a number of menstrual cycle benefits. It minimizes cramps, can shorten the number of days of bleeding, and reduces the amount of blood that is lost. It improves cycle regularity and decreases the pain some women feel at ovulation. Some women's premenstrual problems are diminished as well, and they also may feel less depressed, tense, or anxious. These effects are especially useful for women who suffer from premenstrual syndrome and for teenagers who experience difficult and painful periods that markedly interfere with work, school, and participation in sports and other activities.

Other Benefits

In addition to the health benefits that may accrue from using the Pill as a contraceptive, birth control pills can be used solely as therapy for several disorders, including dysfunctional uterine bleeding (bleeding that is not normal and cyclical), painful menstrual periods, acne, excessive body hair, and endometriosis.

In endometriosis, fragments of tissue that line the uterus implant and grow in other places, including the fallopian tubes, ovaries, surface of the bladder, intestines, and pelvic

SHOULD YOU TAKE A PILL "BREAK"?

During the early days of birth control pills, some physicians advocated a temporary holiday from the Pill at regular intervals, supposedly to allow the synthetic hormones to clear from the body and to make certain that ovulation and menstruation would start again. Greater familiarity with oral contraceptives and their effect on fertility has demonstrated that length of Pill use is not related to future fertility. Stopping the Pill for a few months chiefly results in unplanned pregnancies unless another form of contraception is carefully used. No health benefits accrue from taking a Pill break, and most clinicians do not suggest it.

wall. These displaced patches of endometrium grow and continue to respond to the menstrual cycle hormones by bleeding each month. This condition can cause considerable pain, especially during the menstrual period. Furthermore, the tissue can interfere with the function of the fallopian tubes. By reducing the monthly thickening and shedding of the endometrium, combination birth control pills can be an effective treatment for endometriosis.

FOR THE WOMAN OVER AGE 35

A large number of medical practitioners today believe it is safe for a healthy, nonsmoking, premenopausal woman over age 35 to use low-dose oral contraceptives. "Healthy" means a woman with no high blood pressure, high blood cholesterol, diabetes, or obesity. Some experts argue not only that birth control pills are safe for women over age 35 but also that certain of the Pill's health benefits may have more value as a woman gets older. As women age, they are more likely to develop ovarian and endometrial cancers, for instance, so the Pill's protective effect against these diseases becomes more significant. A number of obstetricians and gynecologists now believe women can stay on oral contraceptives right up to menopause.

In 1990 the FDA changed its guidelines for birth control pills to include healthy, nonsmoking women over age 40. This change came about after long-term follow-up studies had demonstrated that oral contraceptives pose very little risk to these women, and they offer certain health benefits. The FDA also recognized that most current pills are considerably less potent than those prescribed before 1980; hence they are less likely to produce the cardiovascular complications associated with earlier Pill use.

Although a woman may ovulate less regularly, she can still become pregnant well into her 40s. Sometimes irregular ovulation causes periods to be more painful and heavier and intensifies symptoms of premenstrual syndrome. Although barrier contraceptives and IUDs are excellent contraceptive methods, they do not alleviate painful menstrual symptoms and bleeding problems. These problems can last until menopause, which may not occur until age 50 or later. Low-dose birth control pills can be a real boon at this point, causing lighter and less painful periods, reducing period variability, and easing premenstrual syndrome.

Oral contraceptives also may offer a form of hormone replacement for women who are not yet menopausal but whose estrogen levels have already begun to decline. The estrogen in a combined pill can ease the early symptoms of menopause, such as hot flushes, so effectively that a woman does not realize she has begun menopause until she stops taking the Pill and the symptoms become obvious. Some gynecologists believe that their patients should remain on birth control pills until they have stopped ovulating.

WOMEN WHO SHOULD NOT TAKE THE PILL

Some women have a disease or condition that could make it dangerous to take birth control pills. Other women have health conditions that can be worsened by using oral contraceptives. Newer epidemiological studies of healthy, non-smoking women up to age 44 show that use of the Pill is not associated with an increased risk of cardiovascular disease. However, many health care providers still believe that women who have a family history of a heart attack in a person under the age of 50, particularly if that relative was female, should avoid using the Pill when they are over age 35.

Women Who Definitely Should Not Take the Pill

Certain women should not use the Pill at all, and some women should not use it at certain times in their lives. For this reason, the FDA requires Pill manufacturers to include in each package an insert listing the Pill's side effects, warning signals, and other precautions. If you have any of the following conditions, do not use oral contraceptives:

- If you are pregnant or think you might be pregnant. To be certain, do not start oral contraceptives until the first day of your period.
- If you have experienced blood clots in the lungs (pulmonary embolism) or eyes, or have a history of blood clots in the deep veins of the legs.
- If you have ever been diagnosed with angina, a type of chest pain that indicates insufficient blood flow to the heart.
- If you have recently been diagnosed as having cancer of the breast, cervix, vagina, or uterus, or are suspected of having it.
- If you have had any undiagnosed, abnormal vaginal bleeding—until a diagnosis is reached by your doctor.
- If you have experienced yellowing of your skin or the whites of your eyes during pregnancy or during an earlier use of the Pill that was diagnosed as jaundice. Jaundice indicates an excess of bile products in the blood. The estrogen and progestin in the Pill make it somewhat more difficult for the liver to break down bile products.
- You smoke and are over 35.

THE PILL AND SICKLE CELL DISEASE

One of the widely held misconceptions about oral contraceptives is that they cannot be used by a woman who has sickle cell disease, which is an inherited, chronic, severe anemia. Research has demonstrated that women with sickle cell disease who take the Pill are not more vulnerable to sickle crises that occur when the sickle-shaped blood cells block small blood vessels. In fact, the Pill is an excellent contraceptive for these women, for whom pregnancy can be dangerous.

Women Who Probably Should Not Use the Pill

A number of physical conditions can interact with Pill use and be associated with more severe side effects. Generally speaking, the Pill is not an ideal contraceptive if you have any of these problems, but each case should be decided between you and your physician. If you have any of these contraindications and use the Pill, you should be checked frequently by your health care provider.

- high blood pressure
- heart disease
- kidney disease
- family history of early heart attack or stroke
- severe migraine or vascular headaches
- gallbladder disease
- severe mental depression
- elevated cholesterol or elevated triglycerides
- epilepsy (anticonvulsant drugs diminish oral contraceptive effectiveness)
- severe diabetes

Years ago it appeared that *high-dose* combined pills had a negative effect on glucose tolerance and insulin levels. The new low-dose pills have a different estrogen/progestin ratio and seem to have little effect on how the body metabolizes carbohydrates. Women who developed diabetes during a pregnancy and whose glucose tolerance returned to normal afterward can use oral contraceptives as long as their blood glucose levels are monitored regularly. Low-dose pills are good contraceptives for women with insulin-dependent diabetes mellitus.

Other Cautions

Because the Pill can be associated with an increased risk of blood clots, it is best to stop birth control pills for three or four weeks before surgery, for two weeks after major surgery, during a lengthy stay in bed, while a severe injury to a

THE PILL AND VITAMIN DEFICIENCIES

Several studies have indicated that earlier birth control pills changed a woman's nutritional needs. The high level of estrogen prevented the body from absorbing certain B vitamins, vitamins C and E, and zinc. It is not known if this is true of the current low-dose pills.

Blood levels of vitamins B_1 (thiamine), B_2 (riboflavin), B_6 (pyridoxine), B_{11} (folic acid), and B_{12} (cyanocobalamin) declined when high-dose pills were used. When taking oral contraceptives, vitamin C intake can be increased by eating citrus fruits, tomatoes, and certain green vegetables. The evidence is not conclusive regarding the effect of oral contraceptives on vitamin E utilization. Because this vitamin is found in so many foods, however, a serious deficiency is not likely.

Zinc is a trace mineral essential to the body's many metabolic functions, including the action of insulin. Some doctors recommend that women increase their intake of foods containing zinc when they take birth control pills, especially if they plan to remain on the Pill for a long time. Meat, eggs, fish, and milk are rich sources of zinc. Although multivitamins containing zinc are safe, separate zinc supplements are not recommended because too much of this mineral can interfere with the intestinal absorption of iron and copper.

Most women on the Pill need not take vitamin supplements to compensate for the effects of the estrogen as long as they eat an adequate, varied diet containing foods such as milk, cheese, liver, pork, eggs, wheat germ, citrus fruits, and leafy green vegetables.

lower leg is healing, or while a leg is in a whole-leg cast. For the same reason, it is preferable not to take the Pill for at least four weeks after childbirth. If necessary, use another form of contraception.

If you suspect that you are pregnant while you are taking oral contraceptives, discontinue the Pill and use another form of contraception in order to protect the fetus from exposure to hormones. (As a rule, stop taking the Pill only after consulting your health care provider.)

If you are breast-feeding, talk to your practitioner before starting oral contraceptives. A small amount of the hormones can be passed to the child in the milk. Rarely, adverse effects on infants have been reported, including jaundice and breast enlargement; these conditions are probably related to the estrogen in combination pills. Furthermore, combination oral contraceptives may reduce the amount of your milk. (For more information on birth control and breast-feeding, see Chapter 17.)

Do not take oral contraceptives if you have difficulty following pill instructions and keeping to a schedule. Severe depression or a major psychiatric illness, drug or alcohol dependency, or a history of taking medications incorrectly generally also makes the Pill a bad choice as a contraceptive.

HOW TO USE THE COMBINATION PILL

A visit to a clinic or a physician is necessary if you decide to use oral contraceptives. To determine whether you are a good candidate for the Pill, a personal and family health history must be taken. A physical examination, including a pelvic examination, a Pap smear, certain basic blood tests, and possibly a mammogram, are also usually done.

The most important instruction for using oral contraceptives successfully is to take them at the same time every day, in order to maintain an effective dose of the oral contraceptive in your body. If you don't, you can become pregnant, especially if you are taking the minipill.

Read the Package Insert. The suggestions for using the Pill listed in this book are only guidelines. For instructions about the specific product prescribed for you, read and follow the detailed instructions packaged with that pill. These instructions are important.

A Backup Method. Choose a backup method of birth control if you do not start the pills on the first day of your cycle. Condoms, foam, or the sponge are reasonably effective, easy-to-use methods until you begin a full cycle of pills. Always keep a backup method handy in case you forget your pills, run out of pills, or must discontinue them for some reason.

Choose the Best Day of the Week to Start. The most important aspect of any pill schedule is ease of use. Whichever day you choose to start taking your pills will be from then on the day you begin a new pill packet. Practitioners and the manufacturers of oral contraceptives usually suggest starting the

---

WHAT TO DO IF YOU FORGET TO TAKE A COMBINATION PILL

If you forget to take one pill, the chance of becoming pregnant is not great. Take the pill as soon as you remember, plus the pill for *today*—two pills at once—and continue to take the rest of the pills as usual.

If you miss two pills in a row, take two as soon as you notice the lapse. Then take two the *next* day. Forgetting two or more pills puts you at risk for pregnancy—*use your backup method of contraception until you have your next period.*

If you forget to take three pills in a row, compensate for the omission by taking two pills a day for three days and finish the rest of the tablets as usual—*and also use your backup birth control method.* Or stop using pills for the rest of the cycle and start a new pack on your usual pill-starting day of the month, even if you are bleeding. *Use a backup birth control method while you are off pills.*

If you forget to take three pills or more, or if you forget to take pills during several cycles, you probably should reconsider using this method of birth control. Think hard about your temperament and present life-style. Other contraceptive methods may better match your particular needs.

pill regimen on a Sunday, the least hectic day of the week for most people. However, if you forget to refill your prescription and your clinic or pharmacy is closed on Sunday, you will be forced to miss a pill. In that case, it might be better to start your pill regimen on some other day.

Almost all pills are taken in either 21-day or 28-day regimens and come in individual packets for each monthly cycle. The 21-day packets have three rows of pills; the 28-day packets have four rows—three rows of active pills and one row of inactive pills, which are taken right through the menstrual period.

Link Your Pill-Taking with Another Daily Activity. You can remember to take a birth control pill at the same time every day if you associate it with something you usually do without fail, such as brushing your teeth or preparing for bed. Low-dose pills must be taken at the same time every day, to maintain an effective level of hormones in your body. Pill packages are designed to indicate to you whether you've taken that day's pill.

Avoiding Nausea. To avoid the possibility of nausea, take your pill after dinner or with a bedtime snack. Skipping breakfast and taking the pill in the morning may lead to nausea and even vomiting.

Begin the Next Packet of Pills on Time. If you don't start the next cycle of pills on the right day, you are at a greatly increased risk of ovulation and pregnancy. Extending the seven-day pill-free interval beyond the seventh day enhances the likelihood of ovulation during the coming cycle. The hormones that stimulate the ovulatory process increase steadily during the pill-free days until they are at almost normal levels by day seven. If you don't start a new package at this time, the hormone-primed egg follicle may release a mature egg at midcycle. Women who take pills on a 28-day regimen are at a similar risk, because the last seven pills do not contain active ingredients. *Missing a pill at the beginning of a cycle is riskier than missing a pill in the middle of the cycle.*

Keep an Extra Package of Pills. If you misplace your packet or forget to have your prescription refilled, you won't run the risk of missing a pill. If you get the flu or some other illness that causes vomiting, you need to take extra pills to replace those that don't remain in your stomach.

Pills and Menstruation. The start of your pill regimen dictates when you have your period. Your menstrual period usually occurs sometime during the last seven days, after you finish the active pills. You may bleed for only a couple of days, or only have some spotting. The blood also may be brownish in color.

If you miss one menstrual period, but have not forgotten to take any pills, it does not mean you are pregnant. It is not unusual to miss a period now and then while on the Pill. If you are concerned, call your health care provider.

If you do not menstruate and have forgotten to take one or more pills during that cycle, your chances of being pregnant are greater. Do not start a new pack of tablets. Instead, use another form of contraception and contact your clinic or doctor for an early pregnancy test. The early pregnancy tests available today, which test for human chorionic gonadotropin in the blood, can provide reliable results as early as one week after conception, before a menstrual period has been missed.

If you miss two periods in a row despite taking your birth control pills every day, although it happens only rarely, you may be pregnant. Call your doctor or clinic for an early pregnancy test immediately, discontinue taking the pills, and use another form of contraception.

OTHER PRECAUTIONS
Vomiting or Diarrhea

Vomiting shortly after taking a pill can prevent the hormones in the pill from being absorbed into the body. If vomiting occurs within two hours after you've swallowed a pill, take another one as soon as you can. (If you use up all your active pills, take the pill for that day from your extra packet.) If you keep vomiting for several days, such as may happen during a severe bout of flu, use another form of contraception until you have had your next period. Then start a new package of pills on your usual day, even if you are bleeding. If you have severe diarrhea for more than one day, use a backup contraceptive for the rest of the month and then begin another cycle of pills on schedule.

Drug Interactions

The effectiveness of oral contraceptives can be lessened by a number of commonly prescribed drugs. Drugs that affect the performance of the Pill include some antibiotics (such as ampicillin, griseofulvin, rifampin, and tetracycline) and barbiturates (such as phenobarbital) and other drugs for controlling epilepsy (such as phenytoin and primidone). Some researchers advise that barbiturates not be used simultaneously with oral contraceptives; other birth control methods are preferable if you must take an anticonvulsant medication.

Other drugs interact with birth control pills in different ways. Acetaminophen (such as Tylenol and Pamprin), for example, may not work as well in alleviating pain. The effect of antidepressants can be increased in women on the Pill, and the reaction to tranquilizers may vary, becoming either enhanced or reduced.

Obviously, it is important, whenever a medication is being prescribed for you, that you remind your health care provider that you are taking birth control pills. It is also a good idea to remind your pharmacist. Because pharmacists are drug specialists, they may be more up-to-date on possible interactions between new drugs and the Pill.

Certain blood tests can be affected by oral contraceptives. When you are being scheduled for any laboratory tests, be sure to tell your medical care provider that you are on the Pill.

Cost

The cost of using oral contraceptives includes having a physical examination and laboratory tests when the Pill is prescribed for the first time, and later once a year while you are on the Pill. Physicals range from $50 to $150, plus charges for the necessary laboratory tests. The cost depends on whether you go to a private health care facility, a government-funded clinic, or a Planned Parenthood clinic. Clinics that are supported by public funds may charge a sliding fee, which usually means you pay according to your income.

The cost of filling a birth control pill prescription from a physician or private health care facility may range from $12 to $30 for a month's supply, depending on the type and brand of pill and the pharmacy filling the prescription. The most commonly used products cost approximately $17 or $18 for a one-cycle package. Since there are 13 menstrual cycles in each year, the expense of birth control pills for one year is approximately $220 to $235. Packets of pills cost less when obtained from public clinics or Planned Parenthood, and such clinics may offer the preliminary physical examination and counseling for a reduced fee. In some states, birth control expenses are reimbursed in part by Medicaid. Some, but not many, health insurance plans also cover contraceptives.

8

The Pill: Progestin-Only Minipills

The progestin-only pill was developed during the 1970s to eliminate or reduce some of the complications associated with the high-dose pills that contained both progestin and estrogen. Because this pill contains no estrogen and only very small amounts of progestin, it has been nicknamed the "minipill." It is taken every day of the month, even during menstrual periods. It can be safely started a week after childbirth or immediately after a miscarriage or an abortion.

This birth control pill protects against pregnancy chiefly by acting on the cervical mucus, causing it to become scanty but thick in texture. This pill also causes changes in a number of the biochemical constituents of the mucus. Together, these effects prevent sperm from successfully moving through the cervix to reach an egg in the fallopian tubes. In addition, the constant supply of progestin prevents the uterine wall from proliferating, or thickening, and this effect also may reduce the chance of pregnancy. In many women, the progestin level prevents ovulation and also may impair the movement of the egg through the tube, providing additional barriers to fertilization. Like the combined pill, the progestin-only pill produces a spectrum of biophysical and biochemical effects, most of which have not been completely investigated. Researchers believe, however, that its effectiveness depends on the progestin's combination of different actions, rather than on any single effect.

EFFECTIVENESS AND REVERSIBILITY

Failure Rates

The failure rate of the minipill is 2 to 3 percent, not as low as the failure rate for the combination pill. The failure rate decreases with age—for women over age 40, it can be 0.3 percent.

Any alteration in timing, dosage, or consistency in taking this pill is more likely to result in a pregnancy than it would when taking the combination pill. The minipill needs to be taken at the same time every day. This pill appears to have its greatest effect on the cervical mucus approximately four to five hours after ingestion, which then diminishes slightly over time. So it is important that you take it a few hours before the time you are most likely to have intercourse. Higher failure rates are sometimes dose-related, as the amount of the progestin in some pills may not be sufficient for certain women—very large women, for example.

Many practitioners believe that the progestin-only pill works best for women who are not at peak fertility—women over 35 or those who are breast-feeding. Oral contraceptives also do not protect against STDs; for that purpose, a barrier contraceptive is required.

Reversibility

Women who stop using the progestin-only pill appear to return to their normal fertility somewhat more rapidly than women who use the combination pills. When couples have difficulty conceiving after the woman has gone off the minipill, the underlying reasons are often the woman's age, preexisting physical conditions, or a condition that developed while she was on the pill.

HEALTH EFFECTS

Because they contain no estrogen, progestin-only pills cause fewer serious complications and side effects than those associated with combined oral contraceptives.

Possible Risks of the Minipill

Functional Ovarian Cysts. During the menstrual cycle, some follicles in the ovaries do not rupture or disappear but instead enlarge and become cysts. Although cysts do not always produce symptoms, some can cause abdominal pain, pain during intercourse, and delayed menstruation. Women using progestin-only pills are at a slightly greater risk of developing this problem. If the cysts cause symptoms, it's recommended that you discontinue the pill. The cysts usually go away in a few months without additional treatment.

Ectopic Pregnancy. If pregnancy does occur when you are using the minipill, you are at a slightly greater risk than usual of ectopic pregnancy. The reasons are not clearly understood. Researchers theorize, however, that the minipill may not always stop ovulation but may inhibit the transport of the egg through the fallopian tubes. If the egg becomes fertilized but its progress through the tube is slow, or if the endometrium is not prepared for the implantation, the egg may implant in the tube. Symptoms of an ectopic pregnancy— which can be life-threatening—include abdominal pain and vaginal spotting or bleeding.

Diabetes. Although progestins have been known to inhibit the body's ability to metabolize glucose, or sugar, the minipill appears to have little if any effect on glucose metabolism. It is a good choice for contraception if you are diabetic.

Common Complaints or Side Effects

Menstrual Disturbances. Erratic bleeding patterns are the most common side effect of the progestin-only pill and the major reason women discontinue it. Some women taking these pills have no menstrual periods at all; others have periods that last longer or are spaced closer together. Sometimes periods are fairly regular, but there is frequent breakthrough bleeding. Shortened cycles are common. Although some women find that an unpredictable or more frequent menstrual pattern is annoying, generally it is not a medical problem. It is thought that the menstrual cycle is changed because the body's progestin levels are no longer cyclical. Health care practitioners say that the frequency of the short cycles decreases with time.

Nonmenstrual Side Effects. Studies comparing progestin-only pills with combined oral contraceptives have found little difference in the incidence of nonmenstrual side effects. These may include headache, weight gain, nausea, reduced interest in sex, premenstrual tension, and depression. Sometimes these effects disappear after the first two or three months.

The progestin-only pill has not been found to affect blood clotting or platelet aggregation, which plays a major role in blood clotting. Thromboxane concentrations in the blood, which encourage platelet aggregation and clotting, are lower in women taking the minipill, indicating that the pill reduces the risk of thrombosis.

Cautions

Cardiovascular Diseases. Some progestins cause an increase in low-density lipoprotein (LDL) cholesterol (bad cholesterol) and decrease the high-density lipoprotein (HDL) cholesterol (good cholesterol).

Although increases in LDL and decreases in HDL are linked with an increased risk of atherosclerosis, there has been no convincing demonstration thus far that the use of progestins actually leads to a greater chance of atherosclerosis.

Epidemiologically speaking, atherosclerosis is more likely to develop in persons with a family history of heart disease and abnormal lipid metabolism. Because the minipill does not contain estrogen, which is known to protect against heart disease, medical professionals have questioned whether the use of certain progestins might accelerate the development of atherosclerosis in susceptible individuals. So far the answer seems to be no. Progestin-only pills have not been shown to increase the risk of cardiovascular disease.

Health Benefits

The minipill may have protective effects on the body. Although the number of long-term users of this pill is too small to make detailed studies possible, it seems likely that many of the health benefits attributed to the progestin in the combined pill may also apply to the progestin of the minipill. Using the minipill can lead to shorter periods and a reduction in menstrual cramps and bleeding. In some women it also decreases the symptoms of premenstrual syndrome. Because it lacks estrogen, the minipill also is less likely to cause headaches or nausea.

Breast-feeding Mothers

Breast-feeding women whose periods have not resumed generally do not ovulate or conceive, and all breast-feeding women have reduced fertility. Although the chance of your becoming pregnant during the first months of breast-feeding is slight, pregnancy can occur, especially after the menses return.

Hormonal methods are not considered the contraceptives of choice for breast-feeding women. Because estrogen diminishes the flow of breast milk in nursing mothers who use combined oral contraceptives, this type of Pill is not usually recommended. Progestins do not have this effect, and the small amount that gets into the milk has not been shown to have a negative effect on babies. For this reason, if you strongly prefer birth control pills over other forms of contraception, the progestin-only pill may be a good solution. When the baby nurses less often and your periods return, you may want to switch to a low-dose combined oral contraceptive for extra protection against pregnancy and to have a regular menstrual period (see Chapter 17).

HOW TO USE THE PROGESTIN-ONLY PILL

Starting to use oral contraceptives means that a visit to a clinic or a physician is necessary. To determine whether a woman is a good candidate for the minipill, a personal and family health history is taken by the attending practitioner. A physical examination, including a pelvic examination and a Pap smear, is performed. Choosing a minipill is simpler than choosing a combination pill because there are fewer brands available.

Progestin-only pills are taken continuously, without a break. Probably the most important instruction for using them successfully is to take them at the same time every day, in order to maintain an effective dose of the progestin in the body. This is important for all oral contraceptives but is particularly vital when you are using the minipill. As noted earlier, the minipill reaches its greatest effect on the cervical mucus between four and five hours after you take it. This effect continues for a few hours and then begins to diminish, and the mucus starts to lose its protective quality.

Read the Package Insert. The suggestions in this book for using the minipill are only guidelines. For instructions about the specific product prescribed for you, read the detailed instructions packaged with that pill.

Start the Pills on the First Day of Your Period. Take one pill each day until you have finished the packet; then start a new packet the next day. With the minipill you must never skip a day. Your pharmacy will probably let you buy two packets at the beginning. When you finish the first pack, buy another. This way you always have a package of pills in reserve.

Choose a Backup Method of Birth Control for the First Seven Days. It takes at least a week for the full effect of the pill to work on the cervical mucus. Condoms, foam, a diaphragm, or the sponge are good backup choices; no methods that rely on temperature or mucus quality should be used. Always keep a backup contraceptive handy in case you miss several pills or run out of pills, or if you must discontinue them for some reason.

Link Your Pill-taking with Another Daily Activity. Make it easy to follow your pill schedule. Women who usually have intercourse at night should schedule their pill-taking with dinner. If you take your pill at 6 or 7 P.M., you will still be protected the next morning or afternoon—once you have taken the pill for more than one week to establish a good mucus effect. The fact that you must take the pill at a certain time doesn't mean you can have sex only at set times. It just makes sense to have the best protection at the time you most likely will have intercourse.

Vomiting or Severe Diarrhea. The pill may be poorly absorbed if you experience severe vomiting or diarrhea. In addition to taking the pill, use your backup method for intercourse while you are sick and for two days afterward. Take another pill if you vomit a pill within two hours after taking it. If you can't keep a pill down or you have severe diarrhea for two or more days in a row, use backup contraception when necessary and contact your health care provider about how to restart your pill regimen.

Lighter and Shorter Periods. You may bleed for only a couple of days, or only have some spotting. The blood also may be brownish in color. Your periods may become shorter or very irregular. For example, you may have a 28-day cycle, followed by a 17-day cycle, followed by a 35-day cycle. Some of these irregularities may correct themselves after a few months; some may not. None of them is serious.

Breakthrough Bleeding. If you have breakthrough spotting or bleeding, continue to take your pills on schedule. In most cases, bleeding between periods is not serious and often stops in a few days. Breakthrough bleeding is not unusual during the first few months of taking the pills. It also occurs if you have missed one or more pills.

Heavy Bleeding and Cramps. If the bleeding is unusually heavy for you, or if you have unusual cramps or abdominal pain, see your practitioner. These can be signs of an ectopic pregnancy.

If your period is overdue but you have not forgotten any pills, it does not mean you are pregnant. It is not unusual to miss a period occasionally while taking progestin-only pills. If you are worried about being pregnant, contact your health care provider.

If you miss a period and have forgotten one or more minipills

---

WHAT TO DO IF YOU FORGET A PILL

If you miss a pill, take it as soon as you remember. If it's already the next day, take the missed pill *plus* today's pill at the regular time, even if it means you are taking two pills. When you are more than three hours late taking a pill, use backup birth control when necessary during the next 48 hours, in addition to taking your pills as scheduled.

If you miss two or more pills in a row, you are in danger of becoming pregnant. Use your backup birth control right away. Also restart your pills *immediately* and take two for the next two days. If you do not have a menstrual period in four to six weeks, see your practitioner for a pregnancy test.

during that cycle, there is a chance you are pregnant. Contact your clinic or doctor for an early pregnancy test. A blood pregnancy test can be accurate approximately one week after conception. A urine pregnancy test is accurate 10 to 14 days after the missed period, or about six weeks after the first day of your last period. Home pregnancy tests are accurate only if the directions on the package are carefully followed. If used too early, they may give a false-negative result. Do not start your next packet of pills, but use another contraceptive instead. You should not take oral contraceptives if you may be pregnant.

If 45 days have passed since the beginning of your last menstrual period and you suspect you may be pregnant, call your doctor or clinic to arrange for an early pregnancy test. This is especially important if you've been sick or have missed more than one pill without using another form of birth control or abstaining. Discontinue taking the pills, but use another form of contraception until you get the test results.

If your pregnancy test is negative, discuss with your health care provider whether you should have a second test, especially if you have symptoms, such as morning sickness, that may indicate a pregnancy. If a second pregnancy test and an examination by your physician show that you are not pregnant, ask when to start taking the pill again. Without the reassurance of a menstrual period, however, you need to be meticulous about taking the pill correctly.

OTHER PRECAUTIONS

Drug Interactions

The effectiveness of oral contraceptives can be reduced by a number of commonly prescribed drugs. These interactions can result in breakthrough bleeding or even pregnancy. Drugs that affect the performance of the pill include some antibiotics (such as ampicillin, griseofulvin, rifampin, and tetracycline) and barbiturates (such as phenobarbital) and other drugs for controlling epilepsy (such as phenytoin and primidone).

Whenever a medication is prescribed, remind your medical provider that you are taking birth control pills. It's a good idea to remind your pharmacist also. Because pharmacists are drug specialists, they may be more up-to-date on possible interactions between new drugs and the Pill.

COST

The cost of using oral contraceptives includes a physical examination and laboratory tests when the Pill is prescribed for the first time, and then once a year while the Pill is being used. Physicals can range in price from $50 to $150, plus charges for laboratory tests. The cost depends on whether you go to a private physician or health care facility, a government-funded clinic, or a Planned Parenthood clinic. Clinics that are supported by public funds may charge a sliding fee, which usually means you pay according to your income.

Progestin-only pills cost more than combination pills, largely because the market for them is smaller. The cost may range from $25 to $45 for a month's supply, depending on the brand of pill, the number of tablets in a packet, and the pharmacy filling the prescription. A 28-tablet packet of Micronor ranges from $25 to $35; 28 tablets of Nor-QD cost approximately $28 to $30. Nor-QD is also available in a 42-

PROGESTIN-ONLY PILLS (MINIPILLS)

Product	Progestin Dose (mg)[a]	Manufacturer
Micronor 28-day pack	0.35	Ortho
Nor-QD 42-day pack	0.35	Syntex
Ovrette 28-day pack	0.075	Wyeth

[a]mg = milligram or 1 thousandth of a gram

tablet size, which ranges in price from $32 to $50. Not all pharmacies carry both brands; most are willing to order them, however. With 13 menstrual cycles in the year, the annual expense for minipills is approximately $325 to $585. Because even a modest variation in price adds up, it is worth shopping around for the lowest price. Packets of pills cost less from women's health clinics or Planned Parenthood, although not all such sources have the minipill available.

9

Norplant

Norplant combines a commonly used progestin with a drug delivery system that was invented more than 20 years ago. Norplant consists of six flexible, slender capsules that are inserted just under the skin of the inner upper arm, where they can be felt by the fingers but generally are not visible. The capsules are made of silicone rubber and contain the hormone levonorgestrel, one of the progestins used for many years in birth control pills. (They do not contain any estrogen.) The porous capsule allows the levonorgestrel to enter the bloodstream slowly, providing the body with a continuous low dose of the progestin day after day. This technique results in hormone levels that are lower and more even than those produced by taking the minipill. Norplant is effective for five years. It must then be removed and replaced, if desired, by a new set of capsules. Although Norplant is a hormonal method, it has fewer side effects and is probably safer than birth control pills.

With the minipill, there is a surge of hormone soon after the pill is swallowed, but then the level of progestin steadily declines over the next 24 hours. Norplant, on the other hand, delivers the progestin in an unchanging dose. It goes directly into the bloodstream, bypassing the intestinal system and the liver. As a result, only a small amount of hormone is necessary to produce a contraceptive effect. This very low dose of progestin and the absence of estrogen make this a very safe contraceptive method. Like the progestin of the minipill, Norplant prevents pregnancy primarily by thickening the cervical mucus. It also inhibits ovulation. It may make the lining of the uterus less hospitable to a fertilized egg.

Silicone rubber is an inert material that does not cause a reaction in the body. Tubing made from this material has been used safely in surgical procedures since the 1950s. The six capsules containing the hormone are placed under the skin through a single small puncture less than one-eighth of an inch long, using an instrument that resembles a fat ballpoint pen. The procedure generally takes 10 to 15 minutes and is done with a local anesthetic. No stitches are required. If you are right-handed, the capsules usually are inserted in the left arm; if you're left-handed, the right arm is used. The capsules can be removed at any time; fertility returns almost immediately after removal. At the end of the fifth year, the supply of progestin is diminished. If birth control is still desired, the old capsules must be replaced with new ones.

This system of long-lasting hormonal implants began to be approved in other countries in 1983 and was approved in the United States in late 1990. Approximately a million and a half women worldwide have had Norplant inserted. Women like the method because they don't have to remember to take a pill every day or interrupt their lovemaking to insert a diaphragm or use a condom. Although in the United States the

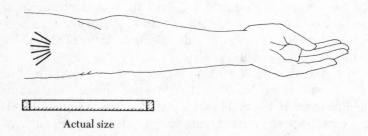

Actual size

Figure 9.1 Norplant Capsules in Place in Upper Arm

expense of having the capsules implanted is higher than the initial expense for any other reversible birth control method, it is a one-time cost. Five years of oral contraceptives or diaphragm supplies cost substantially more. The capsules are almost as effective as sterilization, yet the contraceptive effect disappears soon after the capsules are removed. Moreover, a pelvic examination is not necessary before the capsules are inserted, although one is recommended.

EFFECTIVENESS AND REVERSIBILITY

Failure Rates

Although its hormone dose is extremely small, the failure rate for Norplant during the first 12 months after insertion is less than 1 percent. It attains this high degree of efficacy in two ways: The amount of hormone is always present in the body at a constant level, and there is no chance of making an error while using it. With an implant, there is nothing to forget or to use incorrectly. Its overall effectiveness rate for the entire five years is 96 percent, better than for birth control pills as they are typically used.

The implants begin releasing hormone directly into the bloodstream immediately after insertion. After the first 24 hours, no backup contraception is needed. For protection against sexually transmitted diseases, however, a barrier contraceptive must also be used.

During the first few weeks after the capsules are implanted, about 85 micrograms of levonorgestrel are released daily. Over the next 18 months, the daily dose drops to about 35 mcg and then changes very little.

Reversibility

Women who discontinue oral contraceptives containing estrogen and progestin often find that several months, or more, elapse before they are ovulating regularly again and are able to conceive. This time lapse does not appear to occur with Norplant. Norplant users regain their normal fecundity as soon as the capsules are removed.

HEALTH EFFECTS

Norplant has been used as a contraceptive for more than 15 years—first in numerous clinical trials involving 55,000 women and then as a widely distributed birth control method. Since 1987 a postmarketing surveillance program has been under way in seven countries to learn about any uncommon or long-term effects of this contraceptive method. The study will follow 8,000 Norplant users and the same number of controls, mainly IUD users, for at least five years, even if they have discontinued the method.

Since Norplant's introduction, no serious health complication has been associated with it. Many of the severe complications that were seen with high-dose combination oral contraceptives—heart disease, stroke, and blood-clotting disorders—are believed to be due chiefly to the estrogen in the pill. Norplant capsules, which deliver only very small amounts of progestin, so far do not appear to cause any such cardiovascular problems. No birth defects have been attributed to Norplant use in the clinical trials.

Side Effects

Studies carried out in the United States and in other countries have found that the side effects associated with this method tend to be few and mild, and to disappear when the implants are removed.

Irregular Bleeding. The most common side effects are irregular menstrual bleeding, spotting between periods, prolonged episodes of bleeding and spotting, or no bleeding at all. A period may last for seven or eight days, although the total blood flow is usually less than before. Menstruation can also be exceedingly irregular or not appear at all for two or three months. Some women have almost no menstrual periods while using the implants. For many users, their menstrual periods gradually regularized, either with no bleeding at all or regular bleeding.

Cholesterol Changes. Progestins alter the blood levels of lipoproteins (fats). All the studies of the effects of Norplant on lipoproteins found a decrease in total cholesterol levels. Low-density lipoprotein (LDL) decreased. Both increases and decreases in high-density lipoprotein (HDL) have been reported in the clinical studies.

Headache. In studies of Norplant carried out by the Population Council, 1.9 percent of the women had the capsules removed because of increased headaches.

Functional Ovarian Cysts. In most women, these nonpathological cysts disappear spontaneously. In rare instances, such cysts may cause abdominal pain.

Weight Changes. In the same studies, 1.7 percent gave up using Norplant because of a loss or gain in weight. Weight gain is more common, though.

Capsule Problems. Infection at the site after insertion or the unexpected expulsion of one or more capsules from under the skin, as a result of improper placement, occurred in 1.2 percent of the women.

Mood Changes. Still another small percentage (1.1 percent) of women noticed mood changes, such as depression or anxiety, often severe enough to warrant having the capsules removed.

Other Side Effects. Uncommon side effects include acne, unwanted hair growth, nervousness, nausea, dizziness, change in appetite, and hair loss. These problems may disappear or become less noticeable after several months.

CHOOSING NORPLANT

Good Candidates

Norplant is suitable for almost all women who are in good health. Hormone implants are particularly appropriate for women who prefer to use a contraceptive that does not include estrogen. Moreover, women who have experienced side effects from combination oral contraceptives may find Norplant more satisfactory.

Women Who Probably Should Not Use Norplant

Health reasons for not using Norplant are relatively few. They include acute liver disease or liver tumors, unexplained vaginal bleeding, breast cancer, and blood clots in the legs, lungs, or eyes.

In addition, it is not yet known whether the increased risks associated with combined birth control pills are also associated with Norplant. The conditions affected by estrogen-progestin pills include elevated blood pressure, clotting and other blood vessel disorders, heart disease, cancers, and liver tumors.

It is also not known whether certain other cautions are really necessary for Norplant, because they, too, are based on experience with the combined birth control pills. They should be taken into account, however, unless the postmarketing surveillance program eliminates them as contraindications for these hormonal implants. Even though Norplant has not been associated with an increased risk of heart attack and stroke, you are advised to give up smoking if you use this method of birth control.

You should not use Norplant if you must take certain other drugs, such as phenytoin or carbamazepine, the anticonvulsant drugs used to control epilepsy. In most instances, these drugs can reduce the effectiveness of the contraceptive.

If you use Norplant, be sure to mention this fact whenever you see a professional for a medical problem, and make sure he or she is well informed about the method.

If You Are Breast-feeding

Hormonal methods are not considered the contraceptives of first choice for women who are breast-feeding. If you are nursing a baby, delay receiving the Norplant inserts until at least the sixth week after childbirth. The progestin used in Norplant has been identified in the breast milk of lactating women, but in minute amounts. No significant effects were observed on the growth or health of infants whose mothers used Norplant beginning six weeks after childbirth.

Finding a Practitioner

Although the procedure for inserting the Norplant capsules is very simple, it is important that it be performed correctly. If the capsules are inserted too deeply under the skin, they are more difficult to remove later. The U.S. distributor of Norplant, Wyeth-Ayerst Laboratories, has trained over 24,000 health care practitioners in Norplant procedures. Norplant providers include many trained physicians, nurse-midwives, nurse-practitioners, or other health professionals. You should be able to find a practitioner who has been trained in the technique by calling your local Planned Parenthood affiliate, a clinic that specializes in women's health, or the obstetrics/gynecology service of a nearby hospital.

Norplant Counseling

If you have doubts about any aspects of the Norplant system, do not hesitate to discuss them thoroughly with your health care professional beforehand. Write down questions as they occur to you, before your appointment. Although the insertion and removal procedures are relatively simple, they are not inexpensive, and it is sensible to resolve any doubts about Norplant before the capsules have been inserted. Nor should you be reluctant to contact your clinician afterward, especially about changes in your body or menstrual pattern, if you are not entirely comfortable with them.

The Procedure

To avoid the risk of placing the capsules in a woman who unknowingly is pregnant, practitioners are advised to implant the capsules within seven days of the beginning of the menstrual period or immediately after an abortion. A local anesthetic is injected near the site on the upper arm, an inch or two above the fold of the elbow. A small puncture is made, and, using a special needle, the practitioner places the capsules one at a time under the skin in the shape of a fan. The implants should not touch one another, so that the drug can diffuse easily. The procedure takes 10 to 15 minutes. There are no stitches. After the anesthetic wears off, the area of the incision feels sore for a day or two and may be discolored and swollen. The incision is covered by a small gauze pad and adhesive tape that should be left in place for a few days. Keep the site clean, dry, and protected with a bandage until it has healed. After 24 hours, the implants will have emitted enough hormone to be fully effective.

Because the incision is tiny, it seldom leaves a detectable scar. The capsules themselves generally are not visible. In some women, the skin gets darker over the site of the implant; this dark area disappears when the capsules are removed. The capsules do not move around and cannot break, no matter how vigorously you use your arm. After the incision is healed, you can treat that area of your arm as you normally would.

Warning Signs of Possible Problems

See your practitioner immediately if you experience severe lower abdominal pain, heavy vaginal bleeding, migraine or other severe headaches, visual disturbances, pain in the implant arm, or pus or bleeding at the site of the implant (which may indicate an infection), or if a capsule works its way out through the skin, a rare occurrence. (If a capsule is expelled, it should be replaced.) If you don't have a menstrual period after many regular cycles, contact your health care provider for a pregnancy test.

Dealing with Menstrual Irregularity

Irregular menstrual periods, spotting between periods, or no periods at all are hallmarks of progestin implants, especially during the first nine to 12 months. There is no harm if you do not menstruate; the blood does not accumulate in your uterus. What does happen is that the uterine lining simply does not thicken and become filled with blood as it otherwise would every month, so there is little or no blood to be shed. The absence of menstrual periods does not mean you are pregnant, nor does it mean that you will have problems becoming pregnant after your implants are removed. If you are worried that you might be pregnant, return to your health care provider for a pregnancy test to put your mind at rest. If your periods have not returned after a year, you probably will have few if any bleeding days each month while you are using Norplant.

Removal

Norplant capsules should be removed after five years because at this point they are no longer releasing enough progestin to offer adequate contraceptive protection. They also can be taken out at any earlier time and for any reason. A local anesthetic is injected at the end of the capsules. Removal takes 20 to 30 minutes. If there are complications, such as a deeply imbedded or broken capsule, the removal procedure takes longer. Because they are visible on both X rays and ultrasound, the capsules are always easily located.

Replacement

Your practitioner should give you a patient booklet for noting the date the capsules were inserted, by whom, where, and when the capsules should be removed. (The booklet also has a chart for keeping track of bleeding problems.) A note carried forward from one year's calendar to the next is also a good idea. If you do not have the capsules replaced immediately after removal, use another form of contraception if you want to avoid pregnancy.

The next set of implants can be inserted in the same incision but fanned out in the opposite direction, as long as they don't lie so close to the elbow crease that they interfere with arm movement. A new incision may be needed if the original area was bruised during removal. The implants can also be put in the other arm.

Cost

Norplant implants cost $350. The practitioner's fee, which varies depending on location and whether the procedure is performed by a private physician or in a publicly funded clinic, is additional. If Norplant is used for all five years, the cost averages out to about $100 a year.

Norplant insertion is covered by Medicaid in almost all states, as well as by 33 Health Maintenance Organizations (HMOs), many health insurance companies, and the Civilian Health and Medical Program, U.S. (CHAMPUS), a health plan for retired military personnel and their families. More than one-half of Planned Parenthood clinics already provide Norplant, and this number is steadily increasing as more practitioners are trained in the procedure.

Three

ΛVΛ

The Intrauterine Method

10

Intrauterine Devices (IUDs)

Intrauterine devices—which are small, flexible, and made of plastic—are placed in the uterus in order to prevent conception. An IUD must be inserted by a trained health professional. Once the device is in place, a woman is protected against conception. Only two types of IUDs are approved by the FDA for use in the United States today: the Progestasert and the ParaGard T 380A. The vertical stem of the T-shaped Progestasert contains a small supply of a progesterone that slowly diffuses over a 12-month period, after which this IUD should be removed and replaced. The ParaGard, which is also T-shaped, is partially copper-covered. It is approved for eight years of use.

The advantages of this form of birth control are many. An IUD is extremely effective; it is inexpensive; and it does not require daily attention. The copper version does not produce hormone side effects. An IUD does not interrupt lovemaking, and fertility returns immediately after it has been removed. Furthermore, when an IUD is in place in the uterus, neither partner can feel it.

IUD TESTING AND PRECAUTIONS

The IUD was a common form of contraceptive during the 1960s and later. Many types were available, and one of the most popular was the Dalkon Shield. This all-plastic form of IUD had not been reviewed and tested before it was put on the market—at that time, such devices did not require FDA approval.

The Dalkon Shield was designed with a multifilament string tail, which was later found to allow bacteria to migrate upward into the reproductive tract. By the early 1970s, use of the Dalkon Shield had led to so many cases of pelvic inflammatory disease, infected pregnancies, miscarriages, and reproductive system damage—and lawsuits—that it was withdrawn from use. Eventually all IUDs, except the Progestasert, were taken off the market.

Federal regulations now require medical devices, including IUDs, to be tested for safety, just as though they were drugs. In addition, to further reduce the risk of complications, stringent guidelines were developed by the drug companies for their use.

In 1989 a diagnostic and therapeutic technology assessment (DATTA) panel consisting of 35 obstetricians and gynecologists reviewed what is known about the Progestasert and the ParaGard and issued a report. The DATTA panelists overwhelmingly considered both IUDs safe and effective. When used by women in mutually monogamous relationships, these devices are reliable in preventing pregnancy and have relatively few complications.

Because there is an increased risk of pelvic inflammatory disease when an IUD user contracts a sexually transmitted infection, they are not recommended for women exposed to multiple sexual partners, a history of pelvic infections, or a history of ectopic pregnancy. In addition, IUDs are not recommended for women who have never given birth.

HOW THE IUD WORKS

Exactly how an IUD interferes with conception is still not completely understood. For some time it was thought that its presence in the uterus stimulated a response in the uterine lining, preventing the fertilized egg from implanting. A review of the research indicates, however, that the chief effect of the IUD appears to take place in the fallopian tubes, where it interferes with the fertilization process itself. No fertilized eggs have been found to reach the uterus of women using IUDs. Some studies have found decreased numbers of sperm or no sperm at all in the fallopian tubes of women using IUDs, leading to speculation that the devices somehow alter either the number or the vitality of sperm.

TYPES OF IUDs

Progestasert

Approved for use in 1976, the Progestasert is a flexible, all-plastic, T-shaped IUD with two monofilament threads attached to the base of the vertical stem. The threads extend into the vagina to indicate the presence of the IUD and make it easier to remove. (The monofilament does not act as a ladder for bacteria.) The arm of the T measures about 1¼ inches, and the stem is just under 1½ inches. There is a continuous release of progesterone from a tiny reservoir in the hollow stem. The hormone provides additional protection against conception. The reservoir releases just slightly more progesterone than a woman's body produces in one day during the latter part of a normal menstrual cycle. It acts directly on the lining of the uterus, and only a tiny amount enters the bloodstream, virtually eliminating the side effects that can occur when hormones are taken orally.

After 12 months, the supply of the hormone is exhausted, and the Progestasert must be replaced. It is somewhat less effective than the ParaGard IUD and is associated with a higher rate of ectopic pregnancy. For reasons of safety and expense, health care professionals and women prefer IUDs that can be left in place for longer periods, because bacteria can enter the uterus when an IUD is inserted. The minor discomfort of having the old IUD removed and a new one inserted every year, as well as the risk of acquiring an insertion-related infection, are other drawbacks to Progestasert.

The Progestasert is useful, however, for women who have

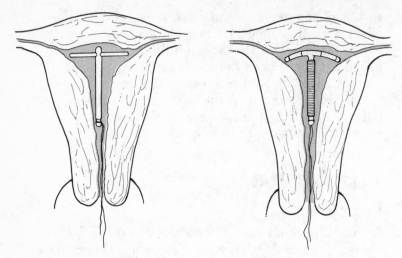

Figure 10.1 The Progestasert IUD   Figure 10.2 The ParaGard IUD

heavy bleeding and severe cramps, because it eases these problems.

ParaGard

The Copper T 380A was approved by the FDA in 1984 and became available as ParaGard in 1988. Copper-covered IUDs have been in use in this country since 1974, ever since researchers found that the addition of copper to the device produced some distinct advantages. Copper IUDs are less likely to be expelled and don't cause as much menstrual bleeding as the earlier all-plastic devices. The amount of copper they shed into the body produces no notable side effects. Women allergic to this metal, however, and women with the rare inherited disorder called Wilson's disease, in which excess copper accumulates in body tissues, are advised not to use this device. The ParaGard is the more effective IUD, more effective than birth control pills, and it has been approved for eight years of continuous use, a real asset.

The ParaGard is made of pure polyethylene. It gains its extra effectiveness from the fine copper wire wound around its stem and from sleeves of thin copper on its crosspiece. Its stem measures 1½ inches; its arms are 1¼ inches. Its monofil-ament polyethylene tails do not facilitate the movement of bacteria upward into the uterus. To reduce the risk of perfo-rating the uterus, the bottom tip of the stem is rounded. More than 20 million T 380s are in use in 69 countries.

EFFECTIVENESS AND REVERSIBILITY

Failure Rates

Both the Progestasert and the ParaGard have been tested in large clinical trials. The Progestasert has a failure rate of 2 percent or less over a 12-month period; the ParaGard has a failure rate of less than 1 percent.

Reversibility

Fertility returns almost immediately after an IUD has been removed (or spontaneously expelled).

IS AN IUD RIGHT FOR YOU?

Good Candidates for This Method

Pelvic inflammatory disease is a possible complication with this form of birth control. For this reason, the best candidates for an IUD are women who have a healthy reproductive tract, are not likely to be exposed to an STD, and have given birth at least once (so that the uterus is somewhat larger). More-over, many clinicians believe that the method is best used by women who feel their family is complete, so that future fer-tility is not an issue.

Who Should Not Use an IUD

You may be advised to choose another contraceptive if you have:

- An active or recurrent STD or pelvic infection, or a his-tory of PID or STDs. (A yeast infection does *not* rule out an IUD.)

- More than one sexual partner
- A nonmonogamous sexual partner
- A history of ectopic pregnancy
- Undiagnosed, abnormal uterine bleeding
- A previous IUD pregnancy or IUD expulsion
- Impaired immune response to infection because of factors such as steroid treatment or diabetes
- Allergy to copper or you suffer from Wilson's disease
- Never given birth

COMPLICATIONS AND SIDE EFFECTS

Complications

Complications with the IUD can be serious, but they rarely occur.

Pelvic Inflammatory Disease. If you are having sex with only one, mutually monogamous partner, you have little or no increased risk of PID as a result of using an IUD. However, if either you or your partner is not monogamous, your risk of PID is higher if you use an IUD than it is for women who use no contraception.

The greatest risk of PID occurs at the time of insertion and during the next few months. No matter how carefully your practitioner inserts the IUD, some bacteria from the vagina almost always enter the uterus, although these organisms usually are not the ones that cause pelvic infections. Furthermore, many clinics and doctors now give an oral antibiotic at the time of insertion to help protect against the chance of a pelvic infection.

Pregnancy. Although pregnancy while using an IUD is uncommon, it can occur, usually because the IUD has unknowingly been expelled or has become embedded in the wall of the uterus. If the IUD has not been completely expelled, it should *not* be left in place during a pregnancy—if it is, there is more than a 50 percent chance the pregnancy will end in a spontaneous abortion. There also is the danger of a severe, possibly fatal pelvic infection or a septic spontaneous abortion, often during the second trimester. Although these risks are rare, they are real. If the IUD is removed early in the pregnancy, these risks are greatly reduced. If the IUD cannot easily be removed from the uterus, a termination of the pregnancy should be considered. When the IUD is promptly withdrawn and the pregnancy carried to term, the baby apparently experiences no negative effects. If you suspect that you are pregnant, get in touch with your health care provider *immediately.*

Ectopic Pregnancy. Another reason for getting medical help if you suspect you are pregnant is to make sure the pregnancy is not ectopic. A percentage of the few women who become pregnant while wearing an IUD will have a pregnancy outside the uterus, usually in a fallopian tube, a situation that can prove fatal. This is much more common among women who use the Progestasert. Women who use the copper IUD have less risk of an ectopic pregnancy than women not using a contraceptive, largely because the chance of fertilization is so low with this type of IUD.

ECTOPIC PREGNANCY WARNING SIGNS

A pregnancy that occurs outside the uterus is a serious medical emergency. If you are using an IUD, call your health care provider if you develop any of these symptoms:

- a missed period, or a delayed period followed by scanty or irregular bleeding
- cramping, tenderness, or sharp pain in the pelvis or lower abdomen, especially if it is on one side or associated with fainting
- any abnormal vaginal bleeding
- unusual pain associated with vaginal bleeding

Perforation. Another rare but potentially serious complication is perforation of the uterus (or cervix) by the IUD. Part of the IUD may go through the wall and part remain in the uterus, or the entire IUD may push through the wall and into the abdominal cavity. In the abdomen, the IUD can migrate and potentially cause a medical emergency. Generally speaking, IUDs that perforate the wall of the uterus should be removed as soon as the perforation is detected. Usually, removal is done by laparoscopy, but occasionally it can require major abdominal surgery. Perforation happens most often at the time the IUD is inserted, and it is more likely to occur when the correct technique is not used or if the person inserting the device is not thoroughly experienced in the procedure. Perforation occurs less frequently if the practitioner measures the depth of the uterus beforehand with a calibrated sounding instrument.

Perforation takes place in approximately one out of every 2,500 insertions. It generally produces no symptoms. A possible signal of perforation is not being able to feel the string. If this happens, get in touch with your practitioner. You should also begin using another form of birth control, because you are unprotected if the IUD is out of place. In fact, perforations sometimes are discovered only because a woman finds she is pregnant. Ultrasound or X ray can be used to check the position of the IUD.

It is recommended that after a pregnancy or an abortion, the insertion of an IUD be postponed until the uterus has returned to its normal, smaller size. Until then, there is an increased risk that the IUD may be expelled or may perforate the uterus.

Expulsion. Most expulsions take place during the first three months after the IUD has been inserted. The body has a natural tendency to expel foreign objects, and the IUD sometimes can be pushed out of the uterus and through the cervical opening. An IUD can be expelled by uterine contractions during the first few days of menstruation, when the os is wide open. An estimated 2 to 8 percent of IUD users spontaneously expel their IUDs during the first year.

It is obvious that expulsion has occurred if you find the IUD on a sanitary napkin or in the toilet. Signs of partial expulsion include you or your partner feeling the tip of the IUD in the cervix or the vagina, pain during intercourse, a string that extends farther into or all the way out of the vagina, spotting after intercourse or between periods, unusual vaginal discharge, cramps, or pain. If the IUD has been expelled without being noticed, the first sign of something wrong could be an inability to feel the string at all. Pregnancy can occur if the IUD is no longer in the uterus. Another indication is a missed menstrual period or some other sign of pregnancy such as morning sickness or tender breasts. It's a good idea to check the string at least once a month, particularly right after your period.

Embedding. Embedding is a very uncommon and usually less serious complication, in which the lining of the uterus begins to grow around the IUD. An embedded IUD is harder to take out and can break during the removal process. In some cases, a dilation and curettage (D&C) or other surgery may be necessary to remove the IUD. Strings that seem shorter may be a sign that the IUD is becoming embedded, and this development should be brought to the attention of your clinician right away. The IUD can be removed and replaced, or you can try another form of contraception.

Side Effects

Bleeding. The most common adverse effects experienced while using the ParaGard IUD are spotting between periods and longer and sometimes heavier periods. It is thought these generally are the effects of the uterus becoming accustomed to the IUD, and they usually diminish over the first three to four months. Sometimes, however, bleeding problems are so severe the IUD must be removed. Between 5 and 15 percent of women have their IUDs removed during the first year because of excessive bleeding or spotting. Heavier-than-normal periods may cause iron deficiency anemia and the need for iron supplements. If you usually have painful or heavy periods, you may want to avoid the IUD, or you may want to use the Progestasert. The Progestasert can lighten periods and reduce cramps because of the effect of the progesterone on the lining of the uterus.

Cramping and Pain. The most common reaction of the uterus to the presence of the IUD is cramps, very much like strong menstrual cramps, as the uterus tries to expel the device. The cramps can last for a day or two after the insertion and may recur during the first few menstrual periods. Aspirin, ibuprofen, and other over-the-counter or prescription analgesics generally ease the discomfort.

Missing Strings. Both the ParaGard and Progestasert have fine, monofilament, polyethylene strings or tails that reach down into the vagina so you can feel them with your finger. Lost IUD strings are cause for concern because they may mean the contraceptive has been expelled or has perforated the uterus. Use another form of contraception until the position of the IUD can be checked. Sometimes the strings have simply been drawn up into the uterus, or they are in the vagina where they belong but you can't find them.

There are several procedures for locating the strings, or, if they cannot be found, the IUD. Your practitioner can probe the uterus with an instrument or look for the IUD with the help of an ultrasound or X ray. Both the Progestasert and ParaGard have an opaque material built into them that makes them visible on an X ray. If the IUD is not in the right place, it should be removed. On rare occasions, removal requires surgery.

BEING FITTED FOR AN IUD

Choosing a Practitioner

Because there is a risk of perforation during the IUD insertion procedure, you need a practitioner who has been properly trained and has had considerable experience in inserting

PELVIC INFLAMMATORY DISEASE (PID)

Women who use IUDs can be at an increased risk of PID, so if you have a history of sexually transmitted diseases or PID, you are strongly discouraged from using this form of birth control. If you or your partner have not been recently monogamous, you are at increased risk for an STD and are not a good candidate for an intrauterine device.

Symptoms of PID include flulike chills and fever, abdominal or pelvic pain, an abdomen that's tender to the touch, painful intercourse, severe cramping, and any unusual vaginal discharge or bleeding. If you experience these symptoms, contact your health care provider at once. Treatment includes removing the IUD and taking antibiotics. If PID is not treated, it can damage the fallopian tubes, leading to future ectopic pregnancies and infertility. Cases of extremely severe infection may require a hysterectomy.

IUDs. Check carefully to find someone who has these qualifications. Because of problems associated with some IUDs and the resulting publicity, IUDs were not widely used in the United States from the late 1970s to the late 1980s, when the ParaGard came on the market. This means there are many health care providers who may not be familiar with IUD insertion. IUDs are inserted by physicians and nurse-practitioners in private offices or family planning clinics, or at state and community health departments. If sources in your community do not offer this contraceptive method, they may be able to refer you to a clinic or health care provider who does.

Before you receive an IUD, you will be asked to read and initial a detailed patient information booklet that outlines the pros and cons of the type of IUD you've chosen. To reduce possible complications, detailed counseling on IUDs has become an important part of choosing this method. This caution does not imply that IUDs are not safe. It is simply that health care professionals now realize that safety is enhanced when the method is totally appropriate for you and you are well informed about its benefits and potential problems.

Your practitioner will also take an extensive medical and sexual history. It is important that you are completely frank about your sexual partners and life-style. You will also have a full examination, including a Pap smear. Tests for pregnancy and for sexually transmitted diseases, particularly chlamydia and gonorrhea, may also be necessary. The physical exam and tests are performed in an advance visit, so that the results are available before insertion.

When to Have an IUD Inserted

As long as you are not pregnant, you can have an IUD inserted almost any time. Your practitioner may prefer to insert the IUD during your menstrual period, making a pregnancy test unnecessary. Furthermore, the IUD is easier to insert then because your cervix is dilated and lubricated by blood, and you are less likely to feel any cramping or to be bothered by the spotting that insertion usually causes. On the other hand, there is a slightly greater risk of the IUD being expelled when the procedure is done during menstruation. Inserting the IUD at midcycle—at the time of ovulation—can be just as easy as during the menses because the cervix is also dilated at that time.

Most practitioners recommend insertion no sooner than six weeks after the delivery of a baby, to avoid the risk of the IUD being expelled as the uterus slowly returns to normal size. An IUD will not interfere with the production of breast milk. The device also can be inserted immediately after an uncomplicated, first-trimester abortion, whether spontaneous or induced.

Insertion

About one hour before the IUD is inserted, you may be given an oral antibiotic and aspirin or ibuprofen. The antibiotic acts as a prophylactic against possible infection from vaginal organisms, and the aspirin or ibuprofen usually helps to ease the cramps that can occur when the IUD is inserted.

During insertion, the vagina is held open with a speculum, the same instrument that is used for pelvic examinations. The cervix and vagina are cleansed with antiseptic solution. The cervix is held with a grasping instrument, the tenaculum, which may cause discomfort or pain when it is first applied. The practitioner then guides a slender, calibrated rod, the "sound," through the os to the top of the uterus to determine its depth and angle. As it is inserted and withdrawn, the sound is likely to cause the uterus to cramp.

The packaged IUD is folded into a slim plastic insertion tube. The IUD is placed as close to the top of the uterus as possible. Then the tube is slowly withdrawn, allowing the arms of the T to unfold within the broadest part of the uterus. The inserter is slipped out of the uterus, drawing the strings down through the cervix into the vagina, where they are clipped to a comfortable length. Both IUDs have two strings.

Before you leave the office or clinic, make an appointment for a checkup visit a month or so later, so your practitioner can see if your IUD has stayed in the right position and if there are any signs of infection.

The reaction of women to the insertion process varies— ranging from none to slight discomfort to a great deal of pain. Most women find the process no more painful than strong menstrual cramps. If you are particularly sensitive to pain, or have felt faint after other pelvic procedures, the cervix can be desensitized with a lidocaine injection.

After Your IUD Has Been Inserted

- *You won't feel the IUD.* Neither you nor your partner will be aware of the IUD, because it is in your uterus and not in your vagina. This is an important benefit of this method. If you do become aware of the IUD, it may be partially expelled from the uterus and you need to call your practitioner immediately. If your partner can feel the strings, they can be easily shortened. You can have intercourse as soon after the insertion as you wish.

- *Check the strings.* The first few months after you've received your IUD is the peak time for it to be expelled. While you are still on the examining table, your practitioner should teach you how to check for the threadlike strings that hang down into your vagina. Learn how they feel and how long they are, so you'll notice if the length changes. As mentioned previously, during the coming weeks check the threads once or twice a week, especially right after menstruation. If at any time the strings seem longer or you can't feel them at all, or if you feel the IUD itself in your cervix or vagina, call your practitioner immediately and use another form of birth control when you have intercourse. Aerobics, jogging, or other vigorous physical activity will not dislodge an IUD. Uterine contractions, often during menstruation, are probably the most common cause of expulsion.

- *Be aware of the possibility of infection.* Although pelvic infections are not common in healthy women who are not exposed to STDs, there is still some risk. It is highest in the months right after an IUD insertion. Since prompt treatment is important, be attentive to possible signs of infection and do not delay seeking treatment if you experience the symptoms listed earlier. Even if something that could be a symptom does not seem very serious to you, check with your practitioner.

- *Watch for your menstrual periods.* If the IUD is expelled or has perforated your uterus, it will not provide protection against pregnancy. If your menstrual period doesn't arrive at all, or if it's late and then is very light, contact your practitioner.

- *Heavier periods are common.* You are likely to experience more bleeding, more severe cramps, an increase in mucus discharge, and spotting between periods with use of the ParaGard. These disturbances are not unusual with an IUD, and they begin to abate after a few months. If you are anemic, however, the heavier periods could exacerbate the problem. Discuss this with your health care provider before deciding on an IUD. If your periods remain heavy and you still want the IUD, you may wish to switch to a Progestasert.

- *If your relationship changes.* If you change sex partners or your partner stops being monogamous, talk to your practitioner right away to discuss changing your method of contraception. STDs are so prevalent, it's advisable to start using a barrier method of birth control immediately to protect yourself from a possible infection. Remember that an STD may not cause any symptoms.
- *Tampons and douching.* You can wear a tampon without any concern while you have an IUD. The IUD is in your uterus, out of reach of any tampon, since that is placed in the vagina. Although douching liquids reach no farther than the vaginal canal, today it is not a recommended practice.
- *Additional contraception.* The IUD is effective as soon as it is in place. As with any birth control method, however, it is always wise to keep another type of contraceptive on hand in case of emergencies. If the IUD string changes in length or you have another reason to suspect the IUD may no longer be in the right place, call your practitioner and use a second contraceptive whenever you have intercourse.

You will notice how frequently we stress that you get in touch with your health care provider as soon as you have any adverse reaction to your IUD. There is a good reason for this. A review of the problems associated with IUDs during the 1970s reveals that early treatment would have prevented many of the serious complications. Too many women who were experiencing discomfort believed it was typical of the IUD and did not get in touch with their physicians. As a result, many infections and other complications were left untreated.

Removing the IUD

The removal process is much simpler than the insertion. The best time to have an IUD removed is during a menstrual period or during the midcycle fertile days, when the cervix is already dilated. In an uncomplicated removal, the practitioner applies steady pressure to the string and slowly draws the IUD from the uterus.

In the rare instances when this method does not work, the cervix may need to be dilated to facilitate the removal. An anesthetic—a paracervical block—can be injected into the cervix to reduce the possibility of pain. If you have worn your IUD for several years, it may be embedded or your cervical canal may have narrowed, making the IUD more difficult and more painful to remove. If the string has worked its way up into the cervix, a long, narrow forceps can be used to grasp it. A forceps or other slender instrument (IUD hook) can be used to find and withdraw either the string or the IUD.

Do *not* try to remove the IUD yourself or even attempt to tug on the string—if you pull it at the wrong angle, you can cause the device to lacerate your cervix.

Cost

The average cost of an IUD ranges from $100 to $600 or more, which includes the device itself, counseling, a physical exam, the necessary tests, and insertion. Follow-up visits may be extra. Some Planned Parenthood and other nonprofit family planning clinics make contraceptives available on a sliding-fee scale. Some clinics accept Medicaid payments.

Although the cost of an IUD insertion may seem high, with the ParaGard this one-time expense provides eight years of contraception. Its annual cost would be less than the typical yearly cost of oral contraceptives, sponges, or contraceptive creams to use with a diaphragm. Consequently, the copper IUD is one of the least expensive methods of birth control.

Four

⋀⋁⋀

Surgical Methods

11

Female Sterilization: Tubal Occlusion

Healthy women may remain fertile until their late 40s, and healthy men are fertile all their lives. Most couples have all the children they want long before they lose their fertility. As a result, they face a good many years in which they have to use some effective form of birth control.

Almost all contraceptives available today have their limitations. They may have side effects, be interruptive, have substantial failure rates, or require much advance planning. As a result, many couples opt for sterilization as a solution. In fact, the most commonly used form of birth control in the United States, as well as in the rest of the world, is voluntary surgical sterilization. Almost 40 percent of all the U.S. women and men using contraception today rely on female or male sterilization. The only other method that comes close in popularity is the Pill, which is used by 30 percent of the U.S. women who use contraceptives.

Female sterilization is more than 99 percent effective in preventing pregnancy and has few complications. The procedure consists of two parts: entering the abdomen through the smallest possible incision, and occlusion—closing off both fallopian tubes. A variety of methods are used to close off the tubes, making it impossible for sperm and egg to meet. These methods are known as tubal ligation or tubal occlusion, or popularly as "having your tubes tied." After sterilization, women continue to menstruate and produce female hormones, and their sexual functioning is unaffected. The surgery does not change a woman's skin, breasts, or weight, nor does it affect the vagina, uterus, or ovaries. An egg cell is still released by the ovaries every month and enters the nearby fallopian tube. The egg cell stops, however, where the tube has been closed, then disintegrates and is absorbed by the body.

Sterilization can be performed with a local anesthetic or under general anesthesia. At some medical centers the most commonly used methods—laparoscopy and minilaparotomy—are performed on an outpatient basis, using a local anesthetic and light sedatives. Both procedures usually take less than 30 minutes. If local anesthesia is used, most women are able to go home after an hour or two of resting in the recovery room. If a general or spinal anesthetic is used, it may be necessary to stay in the clinic or hospital longer, or overnight.

The type of surgery used depends on when the procedure is done, on your health and medical condition, and on the policies and preferences of the surgeon, medical center, and patient. If the sterilization is performed immediately after childbirth, a minilaparotomy is preferred because this approach is easiest when the uterus and tubes are high in the abdomen, as they are right after childbirth. It's called a *mini*-laparotomy because the incision is less than 2 inches long. When sterilization is performed at another time, the surgical technique used is most often a laparoscopy.

If you are overweight, have adhesions from previous abdominal surgery, or have an abdominal abnormality, you are likely to need a somewhat more complicated procedure. You should choose a skilled surgeon and a fully equipped medical center. Although it may be possible to carry out the operation with local anesthesia, general anesthesia should be available in case it is needed. Just which technique will be used depends on the preferences and experience of the patient and surgeon.

The fallopian tubes can also be reached through an incision in the vagina. This method frequently can be difficult to perform, and has a higher rate of complications. In general, it has been supplanted by minilaparotomy and laparoscopy.

THE METHODS

Minilaparotomy

In a minilaparotomy, an incision about 2 inches long is made in the abdomen. Using an instrument placed in the uterus, the uterus and the fallopian tubes are gently pushed up toward the abdominal wall to make it easier to maneuver each oviduct toward the incision. The gynecologist then uses a special hook, a forceps, or a finger to reach in and lift out a loop of the fallopian tube.

The tube is closed off by the application of a high-frequency electric current (electrocoagulation), a plastic ring, or a special spring clip. Some surgeons tie the oviduct with a suture to form a loop and then remove the loop itself. After both tubes have been occluded, or "tied," and returned to the abdomen, the incision is closed with a few stitches.

The minilap is the method favored when women have a tubal ligation right after childbirth. As mentioned previously, this is a good time to perform a tubal occlusion, from a surgical point of view. The uterus and fallopian tubes are high in the abdomen and easier to reach. A minilap cannot be done if a woman is very overweight, however. The extra layers of fatty abdominal tissue require a larger incision, and so the procedure becomes a regular laparotomy.

Laparoscopy

Laparoscopy is the method most frequently used today in the United States and Europe for female sterilization. When performed by a surgeon experienced in the technique, it is extremely safe. Today it's often done as an outpatient procedure, which can reduce its cost.

Instead of requiring a conventional incision, laparoscopy is performed through one or two openings into the abdomen. After anesthesia, one opening is made in the navel. When a second is used, it is made lower in the abdomen. A hollow needle is inserted into the site to inflate the abdomen with a gas, usually nitrous oxide or carbon dioxide, which expands the abdominal cavity and lifts the wall of the belly away from the structures within it. The needle is then withdrawn and a sharp-pointed trocar is used to make a puncture into the abdomen for the long, slender laparoscope. The laparoscope wand contains a light source for illuminating the inside of the abdomen and a lens through which the surgeon can view it. There are many variations of this technique, and your surgeon may use a procedure that is slightly different.

If the operation is a single-puncture laparoscopy, the operating instruments enter the abdomen through the operating channel of the laparoscope. They are used both to grasp and close each fallopian tube in turn, guided by the surgeon's view through the scope. In a double-puncture approach, the operating instruments are inserted in the second incision, while the surgeon uses the scope at the original incision to guide their movements. After the tubes have been closed with electrocoagulation, plastic rings, or spring clips, the organs in the abdomen are inspected through the scope to make sure there has been no injury or bleeding caused by the procedure. The laparoscope is then removed, the gas expelled from the abdomen, and the incision closed with a suture or two. The only protective covering needed for each tiny incision is a small bandage. If any gas remains, it may cause some abdominal or shoulder discomfort, but it dissipates in a few days.

Occlusion Techniques

Probably the most common technique for occluding the fallopian tubes is electrocoagulation. A high-frequency electric current is applied very briefly to the narrow middle section of the fallopian oviduct. The current heats the tissue, causing

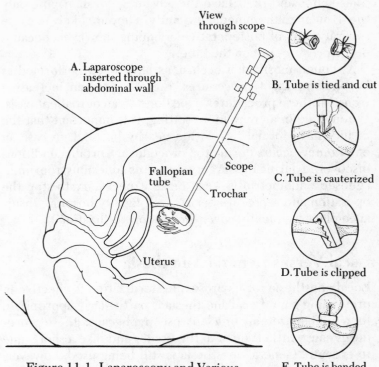

A. Laparoscope inserted through abdominal wall

View through scope

B. Tube is tied and cut

Fallopian tube

Scope

Trochar

C. Tube is cauterized

Uterus

D. Tube is clipped

Figure 11.1 Laparoscopy and Various
Tubal Ligation Methods

E. Tube is banded

scars to develop at the site, permanently blocking the tube. It also kills the nerves at the site, so there is less postoperative discomfort. The safest type of electrocoagulation is the bipolar technique. The bipolar instrument looks like a tiny set of tongs. The current passes down one tong, through the tissue of the tube, and up the other tong, effectively limiting the burned tissue to the area held between the tongs. Unipolar electrocoagulation is also used by some gynecologists.

The oviducts also can be blocked by pinching them shut with mechanical devices, such as metal or plastic clips or small, strong Silastic rings. These devices fasten tightly around the fallopian tube, holding it in an immovable grasp. Eventually the pinched tissue dies, forming a permanent seal.

These clips and rings have the advantage of damaging only the tissue in their immediate vicinity. They are likely to cause several hours of postoperative cramping, however, because of the pressure put on the tube.

Although most tubal occlusions have been performed as hospital inpatient procedures, there is now an increasing trend for these procedures to be done on an outpatient basis. When done in an outpatient setting, it is important that the facility have formal ties with a nearby hospital, in case an emergency occurs during the procedure. Certain conditions discovered during the surgery—such as adhesions from undiagnosed endometriosis—can make it necessary to stop the operation and repeat it later at a full-facility hospital. Insurance plans frequently cover the cost of sterilization.

Local Versus General Anesthesia

Local anesthesia for laparoscopic sterilization is effective in preventing pain. Local anesthesia is particularly appropriate for a minilaparotomy or a laparoscopy, because these procedures cause little trauma to the tissues and take a short time to execute. General anesthesia is still being used, however, because it is the technique with which most doctors are familiar.

Local anesthesia involves injecting a drug into the area being treated to interrupt the function of the pain-carrying nerves, making the area insensitive to pain. You are awake but usually given a sedative for relaxation and relief of anxiety. The use of local anesthesia has several advantages: (1) It avoids risking the complications that can occur with general anesthesia; (2) for most patients it means a shorter recovery time and less time at the clinic or hospital; and (3) it may reduce the cost of the operation by decreasing the charges of an anesthetist.

Epidural and spinal blocks are other forms of regional anesthesia. The nerves are anesthetized where they branch off from the spinal cord. These also can be used for childbirth and abdominal surgery, and some gynecologists now use them for sterilization.

Using a local anesthetic means the gynecologist must make changes in how he or she executes the procedure. Having you awake but sedated makes it necessary to perform the surgery more gently. Furthermore, the physician must be in continual communication with you, telling you what is being done and what sensations or discomfort to expect as the fallopian tubes and other organs are manipulated. Occasionally, you will have to be warned not to move. A local anesthetic eliminates the pain, but you may still experience some discomfort.

General anesthesia, by contrast, induces a loss of consciousness and sensation, usually by combining injected or inhaled drugs. You feel nothing, which helps the surgeon carry out the procedure with dispatch. Nevertheless, general anesthesia is associated with many possible complications: low blood pressure, irregular heartbeat, heart attack, airway obstruction, allergic reactions, nausea, brain damage, and death. Although these reactions are not common, general anesthesia should be used only when necessary.

Each type of anesthesia has its advantages and disadvantages. Discuss them all with your gynecologist. If you prefer local anesthesia, you may have to make a number of inquiries to find a clinician or facility that has switched over to this method or offers a choice of anesthetics. In many communities, however, this option is simply not available.

EFFECTIVENESS AND REVERSIBILITY
Failure Rates

Female sterilization is more than 99 percent effective. The rare failures occur because an occluding device does not work properly, such as a spring clip that does not exert sufficient pressure, or because the electrocoagulation is not complete. A channel can then re-form in a scarred tube and allow an egg to pass through. Failure also can occur if the surgical procedure is not performed carefully enough. (Surgical errors account for one-third to one-half of sterilization failures.) Some occlusion devices and some methods are slightly less effective than others. Nevertheless, the failure rate for each occlusion technique is less than 1 percent.

Reversibility

Never contemplate having a tubal occlusion with the idea that someday you might want to have it reversed. Nor should you forget that life situations can change unexpectedly, and unpredictable events can lead to the desire for another child. Divorce and remarriage, a change in career plans, an alteration in your emotional or economic situation, or the death of a child can create a strong wish to reverse an occlusion. Women under the age of 30, particularly, are advised against a tubal occlusion, because younger women are more likely to experience life changes. Use a reversible type of contraception instead of sterilization if there is even the slightest chance that you might want another child someday. For these reasons, careful counseling is important before sterilization. Counseling is available from physicians and family planning clinics, and no tubal occlusion should be performed without it.

Tubal ligations can be reversed only under the best of circumstances. Reversal does not always lead to pregnancy, because delicate microsurgery is necessary to reverse the blockage of the oviduct.

For a reversal to be successful, the woman should be in good health, be ovulating regularly, have a fertile partner, and have healthy fallopian tubes that were damaged minimally during sterilization.

Some sterilization procedures destroy too much of the tube or remove the fimbria, the part of the tube that collects the released egg cell, making a reversal impossible. It also is not unusual for a surgeon to start a reversal procedure only to find that, in addition to the deliberate scarring caused by the surgical occlusion, the woman's oviducts had been harmed by the adhesions and scarring of undiagnosed pelvic inflammatory disease or endometriosis.

Chances for reversing a sterilization are best if a clip or

Silastic band was used to occlude the tubes. The electro-coagulation method causes more extensive destruction, making it more difficult to reverse. Some clinicians prefer to occlude the narrowest part of the tube whenever possible, in order to preserve the most tissue—just in case the patient someday wants to have her sterilization reversed.

Although microsurgery techniques have made it more possible to reverse a tubal occlusion, the success rates for this surgery are modest, and the expense is high. For reasons of age, irregular ovulation, and other fertility problems, a high percentage of sterilized women are not good candidates for a reversal attempt. Before having such an operation, you and your partner should be tested for fertility, and you should have an examination by laparoscopy to determine the condition of your tubes and whether a reversal of the occlusion is feasible.

COMPLICATIONS

Major complications as the result of female sterilization are infrequent. In the United States, the fatality rate is four per 100,000 procedures. Complications from the use of general anesthesia are the chief cause of these deaths, followed by infection and hemorrhaging.

Complications from the surgery itself can include infection and internal bleeding as the result of an instrument perforating a major blood vessel. Laparoscopic instruments can puncture organs or the intestines and can perforate the uterus. In rare instances, inflating the abdomen leads to a gas embolism, which can be immediately fatal. Electrocoagulation instruments, if not managed carefully, can burn tissues other than the fallopian tube.

The complication rate is less than 4 percent of the laparoscopies performed. Major complications—injuries that require further surgery to repair—occur in just under two out of every 1,000 patients.

After having a tubal occlusion, be alert for such symptoms

as fever, severe or persistent pain in the abdomen, or bleeding from the incision. These could indicate an infection or an injury that occurred as a result of the surgery. Complications can be minimized if they are treated right away, so bring these symptoms immediately to the attention of the gynecologist who performed the surgery. Injuries made by the instruments usually require laparotomy to repair.

The risk of complications from laparoscopy is influenced considerably by the skills of the gynecologist. The clinician who performs any sterilization surgery, particularly laparoscopy, should have special training in it. Furthermore, experience plays an important part—gynecologists performing fewer than 100 laparoscopies per year have a much higher rate of complications.

The most common long-term complication of tubal sterilization is an ectopic pregnancy. Although tubal occlusions rarely fail, if you become pregnant after being sterilized, there is a considerable chance the embryo will lodge in the fallopian tube. Any time you experience any signs of pregnancy, such as morning sickness, tender breasts, or no menstrual period, contact your physician for a pregnancy test. If

ISSUES TO CONSIDER BEFORE STERILIZATION

- Vasectomy is simpler, safer, and less expensive than female sterilization. If both vasectomy and sterilization are equally acceptable to a couple, vasectomy is the medically preferable procedure.
- It is not a legal requirement to have the permission of a spouse in order to undergo sterilization.
- In some states, persons who wish to be sterilized must be over age 21 and mentally competent. After signing a consent form for voluntary surgical contraception, they must wait 30 days before having the surgery.

you develop sudden, severe abdominal pain or cramps, fainting spells, or unusual vaginal bleeding, an ectopic pregnancy should be suspected. Nevertheless, because sterilization fails so seldom, 100,000 women who have had a tubal occlusion will experience fewer ectopic pregnancies than an equal number of women who use no contraception.

WHEN TO HAVE A TUBAL OCCLUSION

From a surgical point of view, the easiest time to have a tubal occlusion is immediately after childbirth, when the uterus and fallopian tubes are still high in the abdomen and easier to reach than when they are in their usual lower position. In the past, when sterilizations required hospitalization, this seemed a logical time for the procedure—the woman was already in the hospital; the surgery did not extend the hospital stay; the operation was easier; and the cost was less. Today, however, most sterilizations don't need to be performed in a hospital, and many women feel that immediately after childbirth is *not* a good time to have any additional discomfort and pain.

Psychologically, too, the worst time to decide to be sterilized is probably just before or soon after having a baby. You may be under particular emotional or physical stress at these times and preoccupied with other important issues—especially those relating to the new baby. The decision to have a tubal occlusion should be made many months after a birth, or at any time when you are able to think more clearly about your life. Although you do not need the consent of your spouse in order to be sterilized, it is a good idea to include your partner in the decision-making process.

A tubal occlusion can also be performed immediately after an induced or spontaneous abortion. Because the oviducts and the uterus are not as enlarged as they are after a full-term pregnancy, either a minilap or a laparoscopy can be used.

Caution must also be raised regarding sterilization immediately after abortion. Abortion is an emotional, stressful

△▽

ARE YOU A GOOD CANDIDATE FOR STERILIZATION?

A tubal occlusion may be right for you if you have health problems that can make pregnancy unsafe, if you do not want to pass
on a hereditary disease or disability, if you have all the children
you want, or if you are not willing to consider an abortion if your
present type of birth control fails. Sterilization may also be the
answer if you and your partner cannot use or do not want to
use the reversible contraceptive methods currently available.

event. It is not the best time for deciding on a method of contraception that is permanent. Don't choose to be sterilized if
you are feeling under any sort of pressure to do so.

HAVING A TUBAL OCCLUSION

Anytime before the surgery, you can change your mind. If
you are the least bit uncomfortable with your decision to be
sterilized or you are not totally certain about the prospect of
having no more children, cancel or postpone the surgery.

Choosing a Practitioner

The most obvious person with whom to discuss the possibility
of a tubal occlusion is your obstetrician/gynecologist. Nevertheless, do not automatically assume that he or she should
perform the surgery. The more frequently a clinician performs a particular procedure, the safer it will be, so you want
to seek out a physician who performs many sterilizations. It is
perfectly all right to ask where he or she was trained in laparoscopy and how often he or she now does sterilizations.

If there are few medical resources where you live, or you
are not satisfied with them, call your nearest Planned Parent-

hood clinic or the gynecology department of the closest medical school or teaching hospital and ask for the names of several experienced laparoscopists. Many hospitals offer this operation, often on an outpatient basis. Some teaching hospitals provide it at very reasonable cost because they need to teach the technique to their physicians-in-training. Some hospitals can offer sterilization because they receive public funds to provide family planning care to low-income families. If you choose a freestanding clinic, make certain it has an arrangement with a nearby hospital to provide emergency backup.

This chapter provides only a general outline—each clinician has his or her own approach to tubal occlusion. When you have chosen a laparoscopist, prior to your first appointment write down your questions and ask him or her for a step-by-step description of the procedure. Don't be afraid to ask questions, particularly about the possible risks of this surgery. If you want more information after your initial visit, ask for it. Sterilization is an important step and shouldn't be undertaken until your questions have been answered to your satisfaction. Make sure you receive the counseling that is a vital part of the process.

Today, before most operations take place, you are asked to sign an informed consent document. In general, the document for a sterilization covers these points: (1) the exact type of operation being performed, including its risks and benefits; (2) the availability of alternative, reversible methods of birth control; (3) the fact that a successful sterilization will prevent you from ever having more children; (4) the failure rate that is possible from this procedure; and (5) the fact that you can change your mind about having the procedure without losing any medical or financial benefits. The last point is important when the tubal occlusion would be paid for by public funds.

Before the Operation

If you are using birth control pills, you don't have to discontinue them for four weeks before a laparoscopy. If you do go off the Pill, however, use another contraceptive method instead. If you are already pregnant at the time of the sterilization, the pregnancy will probably continue unless you choose to have an abortion. An abortion can be done at the same time as the sterilization, but some institutions or doctors may not want to perform both procedures at the same time.

Do not eat or drink anything eight hours before the operation. Take a bath or shower just before you go to the hospital or clinic, and thoroughly wash your abdomen, navel, and pubic area.

Arrange to have someone accompany you home afterward. Because your reflexes will be slowed, it's not safe for you to drive within 24 hours of having general anesthesia or any of the sedatives used with local anesthesia. Your physician will know when you are ready to return home.

Plan to rest for at least 24 hours after the procedure and avoid any heavy work or lifting for at least seven days, to give your body time to heal. Don't expect to be able to work normally, so build as much flexibility and rest into your schedule as possible. Some women recover more slowly than others from the effects of surgery and anesthesia. Often it is a good idea to schedule sterilization surgery for a Thursday or Friday, to gain some extra days of rest.

After the Operation

If you have a minilap or laparoscopy with local anesthesia, you may feel ready to go home as early as an hour after the procedure. If you have general anesthesia, you need to stay longer. After such a brief operation, most women recover from general anesthesia after four or five hours, although sometimes an overnight stay in the hospital is necessary. If you have a tubal ligation through the vagina, your surgeon may also want you to stay in the hospital overnight. If the operation is performed immediately after childbirth, your hospital stay may be lengthened by one or two days.

If you have general anesthesia, you are likely to feel nauseated, weak, and tired until the next day. Your throat will be

POSTOPERATIVE DANGER SIGNALS

Although some pain at the site of the incision and some abdominal discomfort are to be expected, any sign of an infection at the site, any abdominal pain that cannot be relieved by pain medication, or any pain that lasts longer than 12 hours should be brought to the attention of the clinician who performed the surgery.

Other symptoms of possible complications include the following:

- Chest pain, shortness of breath, coughing, or feeling faint.
- Fever with a temperature over 100.4° Fahrenheit.
- Blood or fluid coming from the incision after the first day or two. Red or tender skin around the incision.
- Moderate or heavy vaginal bleeding.

A less immediate—and rare—complication is the failure of the operation and a resulting pregnancy. Because women who have had tubal ligations are at risk of an ectopic pregnancy, at any sign of pregnancy contact your doctor for a pregnancy test.

If the pregnancy is ectopic, you may experience these symptoms:

- Sudden, intense pain or a persistent pain or cramping in your lower abdomen, sometimes on one side or the other.
- Irregular bleeding or spotting, along with abdominal pain, especially if this occurs after an unusually light period or when your period is late.
- A spell of faintness or dizziness (an indication of internal bleeding) in conjunction with any of the preceding. Internal bleeding does not always show as vaginal bleeding.

If you have these symptoms and cannot reach your physician, seek help at the nearest hospital emergency room.

irritated from the endotracheal tube put into your windpipe. After a laparoscopy, you may experience pain in a shoulder— this is caused by the gas used to inflate your abdomen. Although much of the gas is removed after the surgery, enough can remain to cause a bloated feeling for a few days. These effects fade as the gas is absorbed by your body over the next couple of days.

Although the area of the incision is likely to be painful, the discomfort almost always can be relieved by taking a nonaspirin type of pain medication, such as acetaminophen. Take one or two tablets every four hours if you need pain relief. You may have an occasional feeling of discomfort or aching in your pelvic area as a result of the manipulation of the uterus and tubes. This usually disappears after a few days.

Some women experience menstrual problems after a tubal occlusion. These have been studied by several groups of researchers, with conflicting results. Many clinicians now think that most changes in either menstrual flow or pattern after sterilization stem from the fact that the woman is no longer using a contraceptive method, such as the Pill or IUD, that originally had altered her menstrual period.

Tubal occlusion does not protect you against sexually transmitted diseases, including AIDS. Although you are safe from a pregnancy, if you are not in a mutually monogamous relationship, you or your partner still need to use a barrier method of contraception.

Cost

The cost of a tubal occlusion varies, depending on the setting in which it is done and on the physician who performs it. The cost can range from $700 to $3,000. (A high cost does not necessarily guarantee better-quality surgery.) Medicaid and some insurance plans cover sterilization procedures.

12

Male Sterilization: Vasectomy

Vasectomy, the sterilization procedure for men, is simpler and safer than female sterilization and is usually performed in a doctor's office or clinic. A vasectomy takes approximately 20 minutes, is almost 100 percent effective, has few complications, and is permanent.

The term "vasectomy" means cutting the two vasa deferentia, or sperm ducts, that carry sperm—one from each testis—to the penis. A small portion of each duct is usually removed, and the cut ends are closed off. This procedure effectively prevents sperm from getting into the semen that is ejaculated during sexual climax. Although it is possible to reverse a vasectomy, the reversal procedure requires difficult microsurgery. Under optimum conditions the operation succeeds about 50 percent of the time (if success is interpreted as a pregnancy), and it is very expensive.

A vasectomy does not influence a man's virility, nor does it have a negative impact on his overall health. It does not lead to premature aging. After a vasectomy, a man still produces male hormones, has erections, experiences orgasm, and ejaculates. Even the amount of fluid that he ejaculates is virtually unchanged, since sperm contribute only 3 to 5 percent to the total volume. The only change that takes place is that his semen contains no sperm, so it cannot cause a pregnancy. In fact, some men report an increase in sexual desire after having a vasectomy, because they are no longer worried about the possibility of an unwanted pregnancy. A vasectomy does not protect a man against AIDS or other sexually transmitted diseases.

METHODS

Standard Vasectomy

The vasa deferentia that carry sperm from the testicles to the penis can be felt just under the skin of the scrotum. The outer, muscular wall of each duct is thick and less flexible than the nearby blood vessels, which are soft and pliable to the touch. The physician uses the fingers or a special clamp to hold one vas deferens firmly under the skin of the scrotum while injecting a local anesthetic into the skin. (The injection hurts for

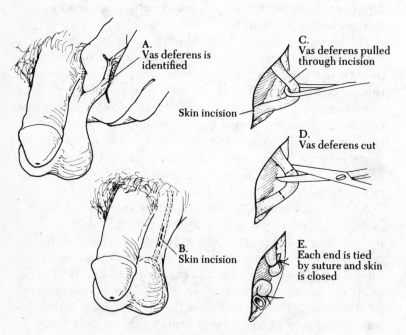

A.
Vas deferens is identified

Skin incision

C.
Vas deferens pulled through incision

D.
Vas deferens cut

B.
Skin incision

E.
Each end is tied by suture and skin is closed

Figure 12.1   Standard Vasectomy Procedure

several seconds.) The new method of injecting additional anesthetic above the vasectomy site to act as a nerve block can be very effective. Anxiety about the injection may have the effect of increasing the sensation of pain.

When the area is numb, the doctor uses a surgical clamp to hold the skin tightly over the vas, making a tiny (¼ to ½ inch) incision through the skin and thin layer of muscle tissue. When the vas is accessible, a very small forceps or other instrument is used to pull it gently up through the incision. Although the site of the surgery itself is anesthetized, you may still feel a pulling sensation on the upper part of the vas. Many clinicians prefer to make an incision directly over each vas, but some make a single incision halfway between the two ducts and draw each one over to the opening to sever it. After each vas has been dissected and its cut ends closed, it is returned to the scrotum, and the incision is closed with a few sutures.

To sever the duct, the surgeon may snip through it with scissors and then remove a short bit of tube to make certain the two cut ends will not join again accidentally. Most surgeons now seal the severed ends of the vas with electrocautery, employing a technique similar to the one used in female sterilization to close off the fallopian tubes. A quick touch of a high-frequency electric current causes the inside of the duct to coagulate and scar into a permanent seal. Other methods include folding and suturing each severed end back on itself, or suturing a bit of the outside sheath of the vas over each end to make sure it remains closed and will not rejoin.

Some practitioners close only the section of the vas that connects with the ejaculatory duct and the penis. They leave open the other end of the vas—the one coming from the testicle, where sperm will still be produced. Leaving that end open allows the sperm to exit from it, avoiding the possibility of a sperm buildup in a closed tube. Accumulated sperm sometimes—not always—can be painful. Fortunately, sperm have a short life cycle. Whether they are allowed to spill from an open duct or collect in a duct that has been closed off, they soon die off and are absorbed by the body.

Such an open-ended vasectomy also avoids the possibility of the epididymis being harmed by pressure from accumulated sperm. Any damage to the delicate structure of the epididymis makes it more difficult to reverse a vasectomy, should a reversal ever be wanted. In an open-ended vasectomy, the end that is being closed off is cauterized with great care, to make sure there is no chance of sperm entering it. Although an open-ended vasectomy is more reversible, it also has a somewhat greater chance of failing.

A vasectomy usually takes 15 to 20 minutes. After a brief recovery period at the clinic, it is advisable to rest in bed at home for 24 hours to allow the incisions to heal. You may experience a dull, aching pain and some bleeding for a few days. You can take an analgesic that doesn't contain aspirin, because aspirin reduces the clotting ability of blood and may prolong bleeding. Men who perform physical labor generally are advised to wait a week before doing strenuous work, to encourage healing and avoid bleeding complications. All men who have had vasectomies should wear an athletic supporter or jockey shorts for four to six weeks to support the scrotum until it is completely healed.

You are still fertile after a vasectomy, until all the sperm that were present when the surgery was performed have been ejaculated or have died. This process generally takes between two and four months—or 20 ejaculations. Meanwhile, you or your partner should use another contraceptive method until two consecutive specimens of semen are found to be without sperm.

No-Scalpel Vasectomy

In the past few years the no-scalpel approach to vasectomy, developed in China in 1974, has been gaining acceptance in the United States. It is termed no-scalpel because a puncture instead of an incision is made in the scrotum to reach the vas deferens. This method causes considerably less soreness, bleeding, and bruising afterward. In addition, the chance of infection or a hematoma (a collection of blood) is greatly reduced.

To reduce pain, some clinicians are using a different anesthesia technique, which is basically a nerve block. A small amount of local anesthetic is injected at the site in the scrotum where the puncture will be made, and then, with the same needle, additional anesthetic is injected near the vasal nerve above the vasectomy site. The anesthetic takes effect almost immediately. When the area is numb, a sharp dissecting instrument is used to pierce the skin of the scrotum and the vas sheath at the point where the duct is most prominent and accessible beneath the scrotum. The same instrument is then used to spread apart the opening. Each vas deferens is pulled, in turn, through this tiny aperture, severed, and closed off according to conventional vasectomy practice. After each duct is closed, it is put back in place in the scrotum. No stitches are required to close the wound. The puncture hole contracts and becomes almost invisible. Antibiotic ointment is applied and the area covered with a small gauze dressing that is held in place with the help of a snug pair of undershorts or an athletic supporter.

A puncture instead of an incision greatly reduces the risk of cutting into a blood vessel. Furthermore, with the no-scalpel method the incidence of infection is substantially lower, and the operation takes only about 10 minutes.

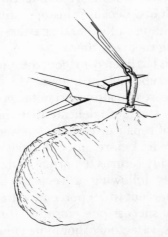

Figure 12.2 No-Scalpel Vasectomy

EFFECTIVENESS AND REVERSIBILITY

Failure Rates

A typical first-year failure rate for vasectomy is 0.5 to 1.0 percent, which translates into a success rate of 99.0 to 99.5 percent. A true failure of the technique can take place only when a closed vas opens or spontaneously reconnects, or when a structure other than the vas—such as a blood vessel—is mistakenly severed and closed off instead of the vas. Such events are very rare.

Pregnancies can occur if you have unprotected intercourse before your reproductive tract has been totally emptied of the sperm that were present when the surgery was performed.

Reversibility

Like tubal occlusions in women, vasectomies sometimes can be successfully reversed. The success of a reversal procedure depends largely on the skill of the surgeon. The diameter of the inner canal of the vas deferens has been described as approximately the size of a pinpoint. To achieve a clear connection between the two severed ends of the vas, the surgeon must use a microscope while rejoining the ends of these almost invisible ducts. Because this operation is major surgery, it calls for the use of general anesthesia, is expensive, and requires a long recovery time.

If the epididymis has been damaged, the injured area of this fine, tightly coiled tube must be bypassed by suturing the end of the vas to the nearest healthy part of the epididymis. Since the epididymis is even more delicate than the inner canal of the vas, this sort of repair often fails. Moreover, it may take months or even years before an epididymis long dilated by sperm buildup finally returns to normal functioning.

Pregnancy rates following a reversal procedure vary widely, from 16 percent to 79 percent, with the majority of clinics achieving a success rate close to 50 percent. For all practical purposes, vasectomy should be viewed as a permanent form of contraception.

HEALTH EFFECTS

Complications after vasectomy are seen in only a small fraction of cases.

Hematoma. The most common complication from a vasectomy is a hematoma, a mass of clotted blood, caused by damage to a blood vessel during the surgery. In most cases, blood drains from the incision before it heals. In rare instances, however, the blood accumulates instead of draining, and within 24 hours the scrotum becomes enlarged and painful. Treatment for this complication may require a brief hospitalization and a longer absence from work. Although unpleasant, hematomas generally do not cause permanent harm. They can be prevented if you spend the first 24 to 48 hours off your feet, preferably in bed. Any upright activity, even walking, increases pressure on the blood vessels and the likelihood of a hematoma. In a review of almost 25,000 vasectomies, hematomas occurred in 1.6 percent of the procedures.

Infection. An infection occasionally develops near the site of the incision. It should be treated immediately with antibiotics. Infections occur in 1.5 to 3.4 percent of vasectomies.

Epididymitis. Acute inflammation of the tightly coiled epididymis duct occasionally follows vasectomy surgery. It is treated with heat, support of the scrotum to relieve discomfort, and antibiotics. Epididymitis occurs in approximately 1.4 percent of cases.

Sperm Granulomas. A painful nodule or lump can develop at the site of the surgery or in the epididymis. This so-called sperm granuloma (a localized inflammatory reaction) is usually caused by the presence of sperm that have leaked from one of the severed ducts. The lumps rarely become painful—only if one touches a nerve. This problem occurs in approximately 0.3 percent of vasectomies. Treatment may require having the vas deferens on that side removed so sperm will no

AVA

ARE YOU A GOOD CANDIDATE FOR VASECTOMY?

Vasectomy is an excellent contraceptive option for the man who is in a stable relationship and has all the children he wants. Men whose partners have health problems that make a pregnancy unsafe frequently consider vasectomy the most reliable form of birth control as well. Similarly, couples who are at risk for passing on a hereditary disease or disability often turn to sterilization—and vasectomy is the safer and less expensive form of sterilization.

If you are young, are not sure about having children, or are considering sterilization in the hope that not having to worry about birth control might stabilize your relationship, you are not a likely candidate for vasectomy. If you are thinking of storing your sperm in case you may want children in the future, vasectomy probably is not for you at this time. (Sperm banking is expensive and not always successful.) Finally, if you have any reservations at all about vasectomy or if you are under any pressure to have the procedure, postpone the decision.

longer reach the granuloma. The lump is then absorbed by the body and stops causing pain.

HAVING A VASECTOMY
Changing Your Mind

Before undergoing this operation, it is essential that you feel comfortable with the fact that a vasectomy is permanent. If you have any doubts, postpone the operation until you are more certain of your feelings. And get as much information on the subject as you can. Other men who have undergone vasectomies can provide you with useful insights and advice. Family planning clinics may do much better than individual physicians in providing information and counseling.

Choosing a Practitioner

Urologists, family practitioners, and general surgeons perform vasectomies. Your own family practitioner or your partner's gynecologist is a good place to start making inquiries. In addition, most hospitals have at least one physician on staff— usually a urologist—who is experienced in this procedure. If medical resources are scarce in your area, get in touch with a local family planning clinic, Visiting Nurse Association, health department, or county medical society. (Family planning clinics often are listed in the Yellow Pages.) Or contact the Association for Voluntary Surgical Contraception, 79 Madison Avenue, New York, NY 10016 (212-561-8000). The association is an especially helpful resource if you are interested in the no-scalpel vasectomy.

Vasectomies and Pain

No matter which technique is used, some men find vasectomy painful. Before the surgery, make sure you understand exactly how your physician plans to perform the procedure and what will be done to minimize the possibility of discomfort. Pain tends to be magnified when it's unexpected, so knowing every detail of the operation goes a long way toward making the surgery more comfortable. A sedative beforehand also makes things easier. As mentioned earlier, an additional injection of anesthetic above the site of the incision or puncture may be more effective in blocking the transmission of pain along the vasal nerve. This subject is worth discussing with your doctor.

Before the Operation

Your doctor conducts a physical examination beforehand that takes into account the existence of any local infections, hernias, and the present condition of your testicles and penis. A vasectomy is more difficult if you have an undescended testicle, a hernia or a repaired hernia, or some other abnormality. A health history notes conditions that may affect the surgery and its outcome, such as past operations and illnesses, as well as allergies to local anesthetics and pain medications.

Make arrangements to have someone drive you home afterward, and avoid all exertion for 24 to 48 hours after the vasectomy. Also get an ice pack to use later. Before surgery, use scissors to trim the hair around your penis and scrotum to about ¼ inch to eliminate preoperative shaving. (You don't need to cut or shave the pubic hair above your testes and penis.) Then shower or bathe to get rid of the loose hair. Wash the testicle area thoroughly.

Bring an athletic supporter or a snug pair of briefs with you to wear after the operation (briefs are likely to be softer and less irritating than a supporter.) This will hold the dressings in place and, by supporting the testicles, protect the incision area from strain and discomfort. Your physician can help you put on the supporter or briefs. Even after the incision no longer needs a bandage, you should continue to wear the supporter until you are completely healed.

If possible, schedule the operation for a Thursday or Friday so you will have the weekend for recuperation. The less active you are for a few days after the vasectomy, the lower the risk of complications.

AFTER THE OPERATION

Get the telephone number and name of the person to call if you have any questions later or experience unusual discomfort. Check with the physician or nurse about how often to change the dressing. Gauze pads can be bought at drugstores, or your vasectomist may provide you with a supply. Keep a bandage on the wound for at least three days—or as long as your doctor indicates.

Once at home, spend most of that day and the next with your feet up. Keep an ice pack intermittently on the scrotum for the first day to reduce the chance that the incision area will swell or bleed. If necessary, take a nonaspirin, over-the-counter pain medication. Check your choice of medication and the dosage with your physician first.

AFTER-VASECTOMY DANGER SIGNS

Call your physician immediately if you experience any of these symptoms:

- Fever—a temperature over 100.4°F—within a week after the operation.
- Swelling near the incision that is larger than the size of a quarter, or pus or continual bleeding from the incision.
- Pain in the area of the incision or in the scrotum that gets worse or doesn't go away within a day or two.

If you cannot reach your doctor, go to a hospital emergency room.

It is normal to have some pain, swelling, and discoloration in the immediate area of the incision for a few days, or sometimes longer. A small amount of blood or clear fluid may ooze from the incision for a day or two. The dressing will absorb blood and fluid and protect the area from irritation from your clothing. If a single pad doesn't seem to be protective enough, use several. If these symptoms grow worse, get in touch with the vasectomist or your regular physician.

To keep the incision dry for the first couple of days, do not shower or take a bath. When you do bathe, wash the incision area gently but thoroughly. If the suturing material used to close the incision is the absorbable type, you do not have to have the stitches removed. If the sutures are not absorbable, you need an appointment to have them removed.

SEXUAL INTERCOURSE

The rule for having intercourse after a vasectomy is to wait until it feels comfortable, anywhere from a few days to a week or two. If your scrotum is still sore, you can reduce the vigor of your lovemaking. Some men also notice new sensations, especially in the scrotum, as testicular fluid and sperm begin to build up behind the surgical obstruction before being absorbed by the body. After the operation there is still stored-up sperm in the semen for some time, so you or your partner need to use some kind of birth control until at least two tests of your semen show no sperm are present.

COST

A vasectomy costs between $300 and $1,000, depending on where you live. As a rule, the cost includes two or three post-operative visits for testing your semen for the presence of sperm. Sometimes the cost includes the first consultation, but often the first visit is billed separately, because a substantial number of men do not go on to have the surgery. Many health insurance plans pay for a vasectomy.

Five

∧∨∧

Other Methods of Fertility Control

13

Cycle-Based Fertility Awareness Methods

Cycle-based fertility awareness methods are based on an understanding of the fertile period in a woman's menstrual cycle and the avoidance of sexual intercourse during those days. These birth control methods are called "natural" because women learn to interpret the normal physical signs of their bodies that signal the onset and end of ovulation, but it is not necessarily natural for couples to avoid intercourse for many days out of each month.

Whether called "cycle-based," "fertility awareness," or "rhythm," these methods are all based on the fact that a woman can be fertile for about 10 days during a typical menstrual cycle. Although typical cycles range from 23 to 35 days in length, with shorter and longer cycles possible, the fertile phase is almost always the same length. The key to the successful use of cycle-based birth control is learning when in the cycle the possible fertile days occur and using contraception or abstaining from intercourse during those days, which can amount to one-third to one-half of the month.

These methods today are known most often by two labels: fertility awareness methods (FAM) and natural family planning (NFP). Regardless of the label, the techniques used to determine a woman's fertile period are very similar. The difference lies in what is done with the information. Natural family planning is generally learned within the context of religious beliefs about birth control, and the couples who practice it use only abstinence to avoid pregnancy. In contrast, couples who practice the fertility awareness method generally use a barrier contraceptive if they want to have intercourse during the fertile days. Fertility observation also can be used to enhance the effectiveness of barrier methods. A woman and her partner can take extra precautions, such as using a spermicide in addition to the barrier contraceptive, during her fertile days.

This contraceptive approach has a few important advantages—it has no negative side effects and costs very little. In addition, when pregnancy is desired, a woman's awareness of when she is fertile can be useful in helping her conceive.

To be successful, these methods of fertility control require intense commitment and diligent monitoring. More training is needed for them than for other methods of contraception, because the signs and symptoms of fertility can differ from cycle to cycle and from woman to woman. Another disadvantage is that neither version of cycle-based birth control protects against sexually transmitted diseases, including AIDS.

THE MENSTRUAL CYCLE

An understanding of what is happening in the female body during the course of the menstrual cycle is helpful in appreciating how these techniques work (see Chapter 1).

The first day of menstruation is day one of the cycle. It actually represents the end of the last cycle of egg maturation and release—the shedding of the prepared endometrium in which no fertilized egg is implanted. At the same time, a new cycle begins: the pituitary gland releases follicle-stimulating hormone (FSH). As its name implies, FSH stimulates follicles of the ovary to enlarge and the egg cells within them to grow. At the same time, the follicle begins to secrete estrogen.

As the level of estrogen increases, it stimulates the cervix to produce cervical mucus in steadily increasing amounts.

The cervical os begins to open. By the time estrogen levels peak, just before an egg is released from a follicle, the cervical mucus has become abundant, watery, and elastic, and the os is open. These changes facilitate the passage of sperm upward into the uterus and fallopian tubes—and to the newly released egg. This mucus also protects the sperm from acidic vaginal secretions. The high level of estrogen also stimulates the pituitary to secrete luteinizing hormone (LH). A surge of LH triggers the release of one of the maturing eggs from its follicle within 24 hours.

The ruptured, or luteinized, follicle now begins to secrete the hormone progesterone. The progesterone causes the os to close and the cervical cells to stop making watery, elastic mucus. In most women it also causes the basal body temperature to rise several fractions of a degree. The temperature remains elevated until progesterone declines, just before the lining of the uterus begins to slough and menstruation begins.

Ovulation almost always takes place approximately 14 days before the onset of menstruation, regardless of the length of the individual woman's menstrual cycle. If the cervical mucus permits, sperm can survive in the nooks and crannies of the cervix for as long as seven days. Eggs can live 12 to 24 hours. Sometimes a second egg is released a day or so after the first, making fraternal twins possible. Women with irregular cycles who want to be safe from conception must consider their probable fertile periods to be as long as 13 to 14 days. This length of time can be a great strain for couples who use abstinence only, rather than barrier methods, for the unsafe days.

EFFECTIVENESS

It is difficult to establish an accurate failure rate for cycle-based methods. They appear to work better for couples who are older and have used them longer. The most recently estimated failure rates range from 16 to over 35 percent.

For couples who use cycle-based methods less perfectly but who have intercourse only after ovulation, the first-year failure rate is 20 percent. Failure rates are even higher among couples who engage in unprotected intercourse during the days before ovulation. Improper teaching, poor acceptability, a high dropout rate, and poor use of the methods are some of the reasons for failure.

For better results, it is helpful to find a health practitioner well versed in this method.

CYCLE-BASED METHODS
Calendar Rhythm Method

The calendar rhythm method was the earliest technique used to establish the fertile and infertile days of a woman's menstrual cycle. It was devised in the 1930s, when it was determined that ovulation preceded menstruation by an unchanging number of days (approximately 14) every month, regardless of the total length of the cycle. Determining the length of the fertile period had to take into account the number of days the egg was thought to be in the fallopian tubes, available to be fertilized, plus the number of days sperm could live in a woman's reproductive tract. This method uses a three-step formula.

Step 1. Make a calendarlike record of the beginning and end of at least eight menstrual cycles. The first day of bleeding, no matter how light, is day one of the cycle. The last day of the cycle is the day before the next menstrual period. After you chart your cycles in this fashion, note the number of days of the longest and the shortest cycles.

Step 2. To calculate the most likely first day of your fertile period, subtract *18 days* from the number of days in your *shortest* menstrual cycle. If your shortest cycle was 24 days, subtracting 18 days indicates that day six of your cycle is the earliest probable time you could be fertile.

Step 3. To calculate the probable last day of the fertile period, subtract *11 days* from the number of days of the *long-*

est cycle. If your longest cycle was 33 days, for example, subtracting 11 days from 33 puts the last probable day of your fertile period at day 22.

To avoid pregnancy, in this example, you would have to abstain from intercourse, or use a barrier contraceptive, from day six to day 22 of your cycle. Your safe period is from day 23, through your next menstrual period, through day five of your new cycle, including days 23 and five. During most cycles, this schedule provides approximately five to six menstruation-free days per month for unprotected intercourse. Many women have irregular cycles, with the result that their potentially fertile periods, as figured by the calendar method, can be long and their safe periods short.

The best way to keep track of fertile and infertile days is to mark them off each month on a calendar. Also continue to record your cycles by indicating the day each period begins. If your cycles begin to fluctuate considerably in length, so that you seem to have more fertile days than safe days, get in touch with the health practitioner who has been helping you with this method.

Temperature Method

Basal body temperature (BBT) is your resting temperature. By charting your BBT for three or four months, you can determine when you usually ovulate. Just before ovulation, a woman's BBT typically drops a few fractions of a degree. After ovulation occurs, the BBT usually rises between 0.4 and 0.8 degrees and remains at that higher level every day until just before menstruation begins.

It is vital to take your BBT every morning before you get out of bed, talk, or take a drink of water. You must also have had at least three hours of sleep. This means you also can record your BBT if you wake up in the middle of the night, as long as you've had at least three hours of sleep. You can take your temperature orally, rectally, or vaginally, but use the same method every time. Leave the thermometer in place for five minutes.

BBT thermometers, designed for reading fractional changes in temperature, cost approximately $10 and are available in drugstores. (They register only the temperature range between 96° and 100°F.) To use the thermometer, shake it down to 96° and put it next to your bed the evening before. If you use it rectally, lubricate the bulb. Monthly charts for noting each day's BBT are available from your doctor or your family planning clinic, or you can make your own.

A change in the BBT of only a fraction of a degree is important. Mark each tenth of a degree with a dot on your chart. Connecting the dots makes it easy to see the day-to-day changes. After you have charted each day's temperature for several months, you will begin to see a pattern. Your temperature changes may be steep, gradual, or in steps. Your chart may contain some unexpected blips that represent a sleepless night or an emotional upset, but that doesn't affect the overall pattern. If there are unusual high or low readings any morning and you can figure out the cause, make a note on the chart to help you interpret the readings later on.

You should see a pattern of one to three low-temperature days before ovulation—the highly fertile days—and then a progesterone-caused rise in temperature. Your fertile period is over after three days of higher temperature.

Because the temperature rise is triggered by the progesterone produced *after* ovulation, this method cannot be used as an advance warning of ovulation. It is an indication, however, that ovulation has taken place and the fertile period is about to end.

Cervical Mucus Method

The technique commonly used today by women to recognize the variations in their cervical mucus was developed in the 1970s by Drs. John and Evelyn Billings, and it is often called the Billings method. The mucus method is useful for determining when *before ovulation* it may be possible to have unprotected sex without conceiving. Recognizable changes in mucus can signal the onset of the fertile period more clearly than does the BBT. *After ovulation,* however, the basal body temperature may be a more accurate way to know when your infertile period has begun and when you can recommence unprotected intercourse.

During the month, a woman's cervical secretions change. The days immediately following menstruation are called the dry days, when women have scanty cervical secretions. These days are considered safe for unprotected intercourse because ovulation is extremely unlikely, and there is no mucus to help sperm survive the acid environment of the vagina. After a few days you may have skimpy, sticky mucus that is white, cloudy, or yellow, is tacky to the touch, and does not stretch. (This very early mucus usually indicates that estrogen is rising.) After it appears, the chances of ovulation are greater and unprotected intercourse is no longer safe.

A few days before ovulation, the body's high estrogen levels cause the mucus to become much more abundant. It looks clear and feels thin, slippery, and very stretchy, and it has the consistency of raw egg white. Some women can take a bit of it and stretch it between thumb and forefinger into a thin strand 3 to 6 inches long. This characteristic stretchability is called *spinnbarkeit.* Spinnbarkeit mucus is also called fertile-type mucus because its presence indicates imminent ovulation and helps sperm to survive and reach the egg.

The estrogen spurt that triggers the production of fertile-type mucus typically begins several days before ovulation. The last day that this type of mucus can be seen or felt is the day of peak fertility. It coincides closely with ovulation but can be recognized only after it has passed, when the mucus becomes sticky again and is less abundant, which occurs for several days after ovulation. From the fourth day after the peak day until the end of the monthly cycle, when menstruation begins again, you are infertile. During your infertile phase, you usually have little mucus for seven to 12 days, and then for a few days it is more abundant, just before your menstrual period begins again.

You can't use the mucus method effectively unless you understand your own pattern. For the first month, you must

LATE OVULATION

Ovulation can be delayed if anxiety, stress, illness, or a change in environment occurs after your last menstrual period and before ovulation. If you then have a peak day that does not seem normal, during the following three days carefully check the characteristics of your mucus. Fertile mucus may reappear, indicating that ovulation was delayed and now at last is occurring. If it's not clear that the peak occurred, postpone intercourse or use a barrier contraceptive.

record your mucus quality every day. Also note the days when there is no mucus. Many women can see their pattern in one month, while others need more time and help from their health care provider or family planning clinic.

When using this method, do not douche and do not use topical medications in the vaginal area that could be confused with the mucus. If you have a discharge from an infection, postpone mucus charting until the infection is cured. When you begin keeping a record, touch the mouth of your vagina every day to check for mucus and make a brief note of what you find. Also note any other physical signs that may indicate a change in your fertility cycle.

During the infertile phase, the cervix is lower in the vagina and easier to reach. It feels firm to the touch, and the os is closed. As ovulation approaches, the cervix withdraws higher in the vaginal canal and feels broader and softer. The os is also larger and more obvious. Look for and record these changes. Also note other signs of ovulation, such as pain on either side of the abdomen, a short-lived ache or pain in the abdomen (known as *mittelschmerz*), breast tenderness, feelings of heaviness, or abdominal swelling. After ovulation, the cervix is again low in the vagina and feels firm and closed. Although you may have no mucus at all at this time, you should be able to detect the cervical changes that offer clues to your own fertility pattern.

Although the mucus method alone can be an adequate guide, many health care practitioners recommend that it be combined with the temperature method for greater effectiveness. A great deal depends on the clarity of your temperature charts and the recorded mucus changes. When several months of experience with both methods demonstrate that the cervical mucus method is an accurate indicator of ovulation, you may feel comfortable using it alone.

The mucus method has several uncertainties, however. It can be difficult to distinguish between cervical mucus and a discharge caused by a vaginal infection. It also can be difficult to tell the difference between mucus and vaginal medications, semen, or the lubrication that follows sexual arousal. Furthermore, if you use a spermicidal cream or jelly, you probably will not be able to observe any cervical mucus. Douching also can wash out the mucus.

The mucus method does have several advantages over the other fertility awareness techniques. It does not require taking the basal body temperature every day. For women with very irregular periods, it requires fewer days of abstinence. And it is more effective than the calendar method.

Symptothermal Method

Because using any one method of fertility awareness alone is far from foolproof, many practitioners recommend the symptothermal method, which combines checking your cervical mucus, recording your BBT, and watching for the other signs of ovulation. The symptothermal method is particularly useful if you tend to have unusually long or short cycles, because the combination of methods helps clarify your cyclical pattern.

You can record your BBT, mucus, and calendar information on the same chart. When using the symptothermal method, it is important to remember that the safe, infertile period begins with these events: after three days of a consistent rise in your BBT; after three days of having a closed, firm, low cervix; and on the fourth day after the peak mucus day. Both the mucus change and the temperature rise must occur before

△▽

ARE YOU A GOOD CANDIDATE FOR NATURAL BIRTH CONTROL?

Fertility awareness methods of birth control work best for couples who are monogamous, because these methods require sharing the responsibility with a reliable sexual partner. A monogamous relationship is additionally important because these methods often involve unprotected intercourse and do not prevent sexually transmitted diseases.

These methods also work for couples who are strongly motivated not to have children and genuinely do not mind the organization and discipline needed to make them succeed. Couples who don't mind abstaining from intercourse and are comfortable reaching orgasm by other means also find these procedures suitable. Men and women who dislike the interruptive nature of other contraceptives or worry about the side effects of hormonal methods may prefer to combine the fertility awareness approach with a barrier method for fertile days.

Women who absolutely must not get pregnant because of serious medical problems that would be worsened by pregnancy and who would not have an abortion are *not* good candidates. They are better served by a contraceptive that has a high rate of effectiveness.

Couples who find it difficult to abstain from intercourse for a number of days are also not good candidates, especially if they do not use barrier methods. Finally, women who are poor sleepers or travel a great deal cannot use the temperature method effectively, because lack of sleep and jet lag can affect the BBT.

unprotected intercourse can be resumed safely. Cervical changes are used only to corroborate the other events.

It's a good idea to record the onset of your period, your BBT, your type of mucus, and your other signs until you are certain you know when you ovulate. From that point on you can use only one method, if you wish.

Since cycle-based contraceptive methods (especially when combined with abstinence) can be difficult regimens to follow, it is strongly recommended that women—or couples—join support groups, women's health networks, or family life education programs. Personal feedback and support from other users of these methods are very helpful, especially during your first months of learning about your body's cycles. Catholic hospitals are one place where you can locate support and find educational groups.

However, some counselors may represent religious groups that do not agree with the use of barrier contraceptives during unsafe days. Women's centers and Planned Parenthood clinics are the best source for counselors who do not advocate the abstinence-only approach in combination with fertility awareness.

14

Withdrawal

Withdrawal, or coitus interruptus, is a method of birth control that requires a man to remove his penis from the vagina when he feels he is about to ejaculate. Ejaculation then takes place outside the woman's body, completely away from her exterior genitalia, thus protecting her from any contact with his sperm. Withdrawal costs nothing, is always available, and does not require using any devices or chemical-based products. Although it causes no medical side effects, withdrawal may interrupt intercourse at its climax and markedly decrease both partners' sexual pleasure. Because it can have a high failure rate, it is best used by couples who are interested in spacing—rather than preventing—births.

Men who cannot control their orgasms and men who have premature ejaculations are not very successful in using this method for contraception. Men who usually produce a few preejaculatory drops of seminal fluid have to be very careful, because one drop of fluid may contain enough sperm to cause a pregnancy. Men who use withdrawal also need very good control and an awareness of exactly when they are about to ejaculate. It's difficult for a man to remove his penis from the vagina when his instincts tell him to penetrate farther. If he starts withdrawing too late, he may leave some semen at the opening of the vagina, making it possible for the sperm to get into the vagina and up to the os.

Needless to say, women often are not enthusiastic about this method. It is not easy for a woman to relax completely and reach an orgasm when she is wondering whether her partner will be able to pull out in time or whether he will withdraw his penis before she has reached a full sexual response, bringing about a sudden uncomfortable end to lovemaking. It also puts the man completely in control of the sex act and of contraception, and some women dislike having to deal with ejaculate on the bedclothes. Withdrawal also does not provide protection against sexually transmitted diseases, including AIDS.

EFFECTIVENESS

Calculating the effectiveness of the withdrawal method is difficult. Only 2 percent of couples in the United States use this method. In a 1990 analysis, the lowest failure rate was 4 percent. But the typical failure rate was 18 percent.

USING WITHDRAWAL

Couples who communicate well and can be cooperative in their lovemaking are more likely to be successful in using the withdrawal method. Moreover, control techniques do exist, such as the stop-start method and squeeze technique, that can make withdrawal more effective and more pleasurable for both partners.

First, during lovemaking, before the penis is inserted, the tip should be carefully wiped off to remove any fluid. (As stated, even one drop of preejaculatory fluid contains many active sperm.) Although experts do not agree on how potent this fluid is, to be on the safe side, remove any moisture at the tip of the penis. You may wish to keep a box of tissues handy for this purpose, for cleaning up ejaculate and, perhaps, for ejaculating into.

A backup spermicide—foam or cream—may have some

usefulness in case semen accidentally enters the vagina or the vaginal opening. Adding spermicide afterward is likely to be futile, however, because sperm move so rapidly. Douching is not helpful, and it may actually speed the sperm on their way.

The Spoon Position

The spoon position makes it easier for both partners to exert some control over the man's ejaculation and can improve the effectiveness of coitus interruptus. The man and the woman curl up together on their sides, with the man behind the woman. This position allows him to hold her closely and to caress her, while at the same time the angle of their bodies makes it impossible for his penis to penetrate too deeply into her vagina.

The spoon position is comfortable for the woman and permits her to stroke her partner's penis and to enjoy his stimulation of her breasts and clitoris. Her legs are together rather than apart, which helps control the deepness of her partner's thrust.

Control Techniques

Two exercises have been employed successfully for many years to help men control their sexual excitement and postpone ejaculation. Both exercises—the squeeze technique and the stop-start technique—require the willingness and cooperation of both partners. Used regularly, the exercises can be quite successful.

The Squeeze Technique. The penis squeeze technique has been employed for many years by Masters and Johnson and other sex therapists to help men overcome a tendency toward premature ejaculation. It can be a very helpful exercise for couples who wish to practice withdrawal because it gives the man greater control over the timing of his orgasm, thus prolonging the sexual pleasure of each partner and increasing the efficacy of coitus interruptus.

The couple may stroke and caress each other's genitals,

including the penis, without penetration occurring, up to the time when the man senses he is about to ejaculate. He signals this to his partner, who immediately takes the penis in her hand, placing her thumb just underneath the glans (the bulbous tip of the penis) and her forefinger and middle finger across the top of the glans, with one finger on each side of the coronal ridge. If the man is uncircumcised, the woman can feel the coronal ridge through the foreskin covering the glans, but the place underneath the glans where she should press the thumb may have to be located by guesswork.

When the penis is erect, squeezing it firmly usually causes no discomfort, although this is not true for every man. Because the response to such pressure is individual, couples may wish to experiment to determine just how much pressure is necessary to be effective. With her fingers in the position described, the woman exerts as much pressure as needed for four or five seconds. (Some women may have to use both hands to be effective.) This should halt his immediate urge to ejaculate. The squeeze technique usually has only a slight softening effect on the erection.

When the man feels his impulse to ejaculate has ebbed sufficiently, which may take anywhere from a few seconds to a few minutes, sexual stimulation is resumed, with the expectation that the urge to ejaculate will be postponed for approximately 10 to 20 minutes.

When the man has developed a certain amount of control over his ejaculation, it is then possible for the couple to go a step further, to vaginal penetration combined with the squeeze technique, to prolong intercourse. They may use the spoon position or the woman may position herself above the man. When he is about to ejaculate, he warns her and she immediately removes his penis from her vagina, employing the squeeze technique to stop his orgasm. This approach is safe as long as the man lets his partner know when an orgasm is imminent. It is important that he not wait until the very last minute, when it is too late for the squeeze to work.

The Stop-Start Method. Instead of—or in addition to—the squeeze technique, ejaculation can be delayed and intercourse prolonged by the stop-start or stop-and-go method. This means intercourse is protracted by completely stopping all sexual stimulation, including penile thrusting, as soon as ejaculation becomes imminent. After about 30 seconds of quietness, the intense desire to ejaculate begins to ebb. When the urge has noticeably subsided, lovemaking is resumed.

Both of these exercises require practice before they feel easy and natural. As the techniques are repeated, the man becomes accustomed to receiving prolonged pleasure from sexual stimulation. He achieves greater mastery over his ejaculation and becomes able to postpone his orgasms for long periods.

As a couple uses these exercises to help the man develop more control of his sexual performance, the woman may also have to find when she is most stimulated to having an orgasm. In the beginning, it may be safer for her to have her orgasm before or after her partner approaches his climax, so she can assist in the withdrawal technique. As he gains more control over his sexual excitement so that sexual stimulation for both of them can be drawn out, the woman may have more time in which to reach her climax. With practice, each partner may be able to have more than one orgasm and still practice withdrawal effectively.

15

Morning-After Contraception

No contraceptive works perfectly. In typical use, many of them have substantial failure rates. And even when methods are consistently and carefully used, accidents happen. Condoms break, diaphragms and cervical caps move out of place, pills are forgotten, and spermicides sometimes fail. Intercourse may occur spontaneously, or a woman may be sexually assaulted.

If the unprotected intercourse was a single event and you act quickly, postcoital, or morning-after, contraception can help prevent pregnancy. The treatment is neither complicated nor expensive. But it must be started within 72 hours—preferably sooner—after the act of intercourse took place. *The sooner treatment begins, the greater its chance of success.*

When you request morning-after contraception, the first important assessment is whether intercourse took place during the fertile days of your menstrual cycle. Most practitioners feel that morning-after treatment is not necessary if intercourse did not coincide with the time of ovulation (at the midpoint of the menstrual cycle). Women with irregular cycles may have difficulty calculating the time of ovulation, and, for them, postcoital contraception may be sensible if unprotected intercourse took place at other times during the cycle as well.

Although several methods of morning-after contraception

have been employed in the past, today only one is in common use. Sometimes called the Yuzpe regimen, it consists of taking two tablets of a combined oral contraceptive as soon as possible after a single act of unprotected intercourse. This dose is followed by two more tablets 12 hours later. Each tablet should contain 50 micrograms of a synthetic estrogen and 0.5 milligrams of synthetic progestin. The total amount of hormones taken in this regimen—200 mcg of estrogen and 2 mg of progestin—is fairly low, yet it alters the lining of the uterus and prevents the implantation of a fertilized egg.

The effectiveness of this treatment is extremely time-dependent—the sooner after intercourse the pills are taken, the more likely it is to be effective. If more than 72 hours pass before you seek postcoital contraception, it is likely that the fertilized egg will have already reached the uterus and begun the implantation process. For morning-after contraception to work, the endometrium must be altered *before* the fertilized egg reaches the uterus.

EFFECTIVENESS

The Yuzpe regimen was tested on 1,300 Canadian women, with a pregnancy rate of 0.16 to 1.6 percent. Almost all the women began a menstrual period within 21 days of the treatment. A smaller study in California of 115 university women experienced no failures, and the majority of the women began menstruating within 30 days. The efficacy of the regimen may be affected by the same medications that lessen the effect of birth control pills (see Chapter 7). The Yuzpe method is also less effective in women who are very overweight.

HEALTH EFFECTS

The side effects associated with morning-after contraception are similar to those associated with any combined oral contraceptive. For example, you may experience some nausea for a day or two. Some physicians and clinics automatically provide an antinausea suppository to use in case of vomiting. Use the antinausea medications only when necessary, particularly if you may be pregnant, because of the theoretical possibility that if the treatment doesn't succeed and the pregnancy is carried to term, the drugs may harm the fetus. Extra pills are usually provided in case the tablets are vomited in the first hour.

More Serious Complications

It is highly unlikely that consuming only four birth control pills will cause hormone-related complications. But to be on the safe side, most practitioners routinely ask their patients to watch for the danger signals that are associated with combined birth control pills—severe chest pain, cough, or shortness of breath; severe headache; dizziness; a feeling of weakness or numbness; vision loss or blurring; severe pain or cramp in the thigh or calf of the leg. Complications are most likely to be experienced within two weeks after taking the pills.

Another health issue associated with combined pills is their possible effect if the treatment doesn't succeed and you become pregnant and decide to carry the pregnancy to term. The Yuzpe regimen for postcoital contraception has been in use since the mid-1970s, and the only complication it has been found to cause is nausea and vomiting. Because the pills are largely metabolized before the egg has anchored in the uterus and implanted, there is no danger of fetal malformations.

Factors that may make it dangerous to use this brief regimen of combined oral contraceptives include smoking or a history of blood-clotting problems, stroke, and heart attack. When these conditions exist, the woman seeking postcoital contraception should be carefully evaluated by her health care provider.

OTHER MORNING-AFTER METHODS
Diethylstilbestrol (DES)

Diethylstilbestrol, or DES, was one of the first estrogens synthesized in a laboratory; it became available for medical purposes in the 1940s. Thirty years later, however, a connection was found between the use of DES during pregnancy (supposedly to prevent miscarriage) and structural abnormalities and rare cancers in the reproductive systems of offspring. As a result, in the United States DES is no longer used in pregnant women or for postcoital contraception.

Intrauterine Devices

At one time, insertion of a copper-covered IUD within seven days of a single act of unprotected intercourse also was employed to prevent a pregnancy. But because STDs are now so common, it often is not safe to insert an IUD without testing for these infections beforehand, particularly for chlamydia and gonorrhea. This makes an IUD a less practical method for morning-after contraception.

Menstrual Extraction

In menstrual extraction, a narrow plastic tube is inserted into the uterus, and then suction is applied to the outer end to draw out the entire endometrium. This procedure must be done thoroughly to be successful. Menstrual extraction is similar to the vacuum aspiration abortion procedure performed during the first trimester of pregnancy (see Chapter 16).

Extraction can be performed up to two weeks after a missed menstrual period. However, if you seek help more than 72 hours after unprotected intercourse, you are usually advised to wait and see if you get your period. If it does not appear and a urine test indicates pregnancy, then an early abortion is usually recommended as a more appropriate procedure.

USING MORNING-AFTER CONTRACEPTION

Finding a Clinic or Practitioner

Many women's health centers and family planning clinics, including Planned Parenthood clinics, provide birth control pills for morning-after contraception. (Many family physicians and gynecologists are less willing to offer this service.)

Because this treatment is successful only if started within 72 hours after the unprotected intercourse, it is important to find assistance immediately. It is best to do so by telephone, because clinics generally prefer to determine beforehand whether you are truly at risk for a pregnancy and are a good candidate for morning-after protection. Expect to answer the following questions:

- What was the date of your last menstrual period?
- Was it a normal period?
- On what date and at what time did the unprotected intercourse occur?
- Have you had unprotected intercourse at any other time since your last period?
- Do you have a history of smoking, blood clotting problems, heart disease, stroke, inflammation of the veins such as phlebitis, or cancer of the uterus, cervix, vagina, or breasts?

Telephone screening saves vital time in scheduling you for postcoital contraception or when referring you to another source of care, which sometimes is necessary. If you have serious health problems, for example, you almost always will be told to see a private physician for postcoital pregnancy prevention. If you call a clinic because you were raped, you will probably be referred to the nearest rape crisis center or the emergency room of the local hospital. Rape is a criminal act, and rape centers are trained to gather evidence and deal with the other legal issues involved, as well as to provide care and counseling.

You should be aware that some antiabortion groups advertise in the Yellow Pages as "family planning centers" or abortion providers. If they offer pregnancy testing, they may delay your test or discourage you from using morning-after contraception.

If you are a candidate for morning-after treatment, a legitimate clinic will schedule you to be seen as soon as possible. If the clinic you called cannot fit you into its schedule or does not supply morning-after care, ask for a referral to another source.

As mentioned previously, if the unprotected intercourse took place during the nonfertile days of the month, health care providers generally suggest that you wait and see whether you menstruate on schedule. If menstruation does not occur, make an appointment for a pregnancy test. The chance of conception taking place during the safe days of a cycle is relatively small after a single act of unprotected intercourse.

THE MORNING-AFTER TREATMENT

A physical examination is part of morning-after pregnancy prevention. It usually includes a pelvic examination, the urine pregnancy test (to make sure you are not already pregnant), a blood pressure check, and possibly tests for STDs. You will also be asked to read and sign an informed consent form. Along with the birth control pills, you receive an emergency telephone number if you experience any health effects or other problems. If an emergency number is not automatically supplied, ask for it. It is sensible that you watch for symptoms of complications for at least two weeks after taking the hormone treatment.

You will be given the pills and will probably be told to take the first two at the clinic. The sooner the hormones enter your bloodstream, the greater the likelihood that the treatment will be effective. You take two more pills 12 hours after the first dose. If you experience nausea, it may be very mild and disappear by the next day. If you vomit within 60 minutes of taking the pills, however, use the antinausea medication supplied by the clinic and then take any extra pills you were given. Follow them with the final two pills 12 hours later. If you were not given any antinausea medication, report the nausea and vomiting to the clinician who treated you. A prescription for this medication can be telephoned to your nearest pharmacy during business hours. (If you live at some distance from the clinic or from a drugstore, explain this to clinic personnel. It may be possible to supply you with antinausea medication before you leave.)

Afterward

Your next menstrual period should begin sometime within the next few weeks. If your period has not begun by the three-week mark, see your practitioner for an examination and pregnancy test. Many clinics routinely schedule their clients for a follow-up check and a pregnancy test three weeks after they have been treated, to make certain their menstrual period was normal. The failure rate for this pregnancy intervention technique is very low, but because the pills act chiefly on the lining of the uterus, they may have no effect on an ectopic (tubal) pregnancy. If your menstruation was not completely normal after treatment, it's necessary to rule out the possibility of a tubal pregnancy.

COST

The cost of morning-after contraception depends a great deal on where it is obtained. Planned Parenthood and other clinics make this service available at fees ranging from $35 to $70 for the physical examination, the pregnancy test, and the pills. The fee for a follow-up visit is usually limited to the cost of the pregnancy test; clinics usually charge approximately $10 to $20 for the early pregnancy test.

MORNING-AFTER PROTECTION FOLLOWING RAPE

If you have been the victim of a sexual assault, seek care immediately. Because of the urgent need for counseling, the danger of having been exposed to an STD (including AIDS), and the fact that rape is a criminal act that should be reported to the police, the best care is found at a hospital-based rape crisis center. You can often locate these centers by calling your family physician, the police or health department, or the nearest hospital. If there is no such center in your community, the emergency room of the local hospital may have health care workers trained to handle this sort of emergency. If none is available, seek care at a family planning clinic, at a women's health center, or from a sympathetic private physician. Or call the Planned Parenthood clinic in the nearest large city for assistance.

At a rape crisis center, you will be given a physical examination. Information is gathered on the sex acts performed, whether ejaculation took place, what sort of contraception you are using, and where you are in your menstrual cycle. A pregnancy test is performed to rule out the possibility of an earlier, unknown pregnancy from consensual intercourse. If you are not already pregnant, are at risk for pregnancy from the rape, and 72 hours have not elapsed since the rape, you are treated with combined oral contraceptives. If more than 72 hours have passed, you are advised to return to the center for a blood early pregnancy test about a week before your period would normally occur. It's possible that the stress of the assault is likely to make your period late, even if you are not pregnant.

In addition to furnishing protection against pregnancy, clinicians take blood and vaginal samples for testing for gonorrhea, chlamydia, and syphilis. Preventive protection against these three STDs is provided by giving you both tetracycline and penicillin. You will also be counseled on how to deal with the possibility that you may have been infected with herpes and AIDS.

As part of the physical examination, evidence of the assault is collected. It is sent to the police crime laboratory and filed there in the event the rapist is caught and you wish to have him prosecuted. In most cases, the evidence is identified by number rather than name, in order to protect your privacy.

Private practitioners are likely to charge $75 to $150 for postcoital contraception. The bill for a follow-up pregnancy test by a private physician will include the cost of the visit as well as the cost of the test.

Six

∧∨∧

Other Issues in Birth Control

16

Abortion

A woman is fertile for about 30 years of her life span. If she has a normal reproductive system, becomes sexually active in her teens, and uses no contraception, she could bear more than a dozen children during her lifetime. As a result, for much of her reproductive life the average woman is trying either to postpone or to avoid pregnancy.

More than half the 6 million pregnancies that occur in the United States each year are unintended. Of these, about 1.6 million are ended by an induced abortion. By the time they reach menopause, two-thirds of American women have had at least one unintended pregnancy, and many have had an abortion. (Strictly speaking, abortion is not a method of contraception because it is not used to *prevent* conception but to terminate an unwanted pregnancy. Most women would prefer to prevent conception rather than use abortion to control their fertility.)

According to researchers at the Alan Guttmacher Institute, 92 percent of fertile women use some form of contraception. But 43 percent of all unintended pregnancies are experienced by couples who practice birth control. (The very small percentage of women who do not use contraceptives account for the remaining 57 percent of unintended pregnancies.)

Almost all abortions take place between the seventh and

thirteenth weeks of gestation, in the first trimester of a pregnancy. Abortions are not done before the sixth week because
the embryo is too small to find easily. About one-half are carried out before the eighth week. Abortions during the sixth
to eighth week are the safest and easiest to perform and
are available as outpatient procedures. The method most
frequently used is vacuum aspiration, also called suction
curettage.

After the thirteenth week, the pregnancy is in the second
trimester. The method used to end a pregnancy now is dilation and evacuation, termed a D&E. As each additional week
of pregnancy passes, the risk of complications increases. In
addition, after the thirteenth week the cost increases as the
pregnancy advances. Very few abortions take place after 20
weeks.

Although some abortions are performed in hospitals, the
majority are carried out in clinics as outpatient procedures.
Most clinics limit their services to the early months of pregnancy. (Only 25 percent of abortion providers perform abortions after the sixteenth week of pregnancy, and then usually
because it is medically indicated.) In the late 1980s, the office
of the Surgeon General, having reviewed more than 250

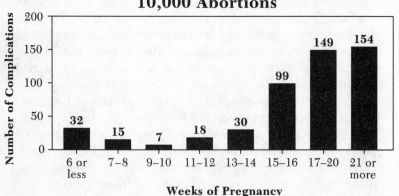

**Serious Complications for Every
10,000 Abortions**

Source: F.H. Stewart and F.J. Guest, et al. *Understanding Your Body*. New York:
Bantam, 1987.

studies, found no support for claims that legal abortion causes women emotional damage. They did note that a woman's distress is greatest before an abortion and that most women reported feeling relieved and calm afterward, especially following a first-trimester abortion.

HAVING AN ABORTION
The First Step: A Pregnancy Test

You can find out if you are pregnant by taking a pregnancy test. You can test yourself at home with a kit available at any drugstore. These tests are reliable if you follow the directions carefully. If the test is negative but you still don't have a period, you need to have a professional test. In fact, the best first step is to go to a clinic or a doctor for a pregnancy test and to do this immediately.

The early laboratory test for determining pregnancy—a blood test—is so sensitive that it can reliably detect the very low levels of the pregnancy hormone, human chorionic gonadotropin, in your blood as early as seven, eight, or nine days after you've conceived. (A standard urine test can confirm the existence of a pregnancy 28 days after conception, when a period is about two weeks overdue.) In addition to the laboratory findings, a pelvic examination is necessary to confirm pregnancy test results and to estimate how advanced is the pregnancy. Whether or not you are considering an abortion or will continue with your pregnancy, an accurate dating of the term of pregnancy is important. If your physician cannot determine how far along the pregnancy is, an ultrasound evaluation may be necessary. Even as early as six weeks after your last normal menstruation, ultrasound can visualize the pregnancy sac inside your uterus, which allows measurements to be taken.

Even with the blood early pregnancy test, the window of time available for making a decision is small. By the time most women realize they are pregnant, the pregnancy is usually six weeks along. As stated previously, abortion is easier, safer, and much less expensive when carried out before ten weeks.

This leaves about four weeks for assessing your feelings about having a baby, about your partner, and about your life situation.

Ideally, the best place to get a pregnancy test is from a physician or clinic that can also provide you with objective counseling and help you carry out whatever decision you make about continuing the pregnancy. The best family planning clinics and doctors offer information on abortion, or where to go for prenatal care, and, if wanted, adoption procedures. If the test shows that you are *not* pregnant, this type of clinic or health care provider can help you find a dependable method of birth control. *Wherever you go for a pregnancy test, make sure it is understood that you need an immediate appointment to verify a pregnancy.* If you will have to wait more than a few days for an appointment, find another doctor or clinic.

Because it is so important not to put off getting a pregnancy test, if you do not have ready access to a clinic that provides a range of family planning services, obtain a pregnancy test from your family physician or your obstetrician/gynecologist. Although your own doctor may not perform abortions, a pregnancy test is a routine laboratory procedure. If you ask, the doctor may also help you find a reputable provider of family planning services. If you don't have a doctor, the county health department or a nearby hospital may offer pregnancy testing, abortions, or information on clinics that offer abortion. In some cities, there also may be an independent laboratory that offers pregnancy testing.

Finding a Clinic or Physician

In 1991 government regulations barred clinics that receive federal funds from discussing abortion in any way with their patients. Although, as of this writing, abortions are still a constitutional right, doctors and other personnel in these clinics cannot mention abortion as an option, nor can they refer patients to privately funded family planning centers that do offer abortion as an alternative. This decision affects approximately 4,300 family planning clinics across the country.

Freestanding clinics are the most common providers of

abortion services. Because many abortions are performed in these facilities, the attending physicians are extremely skilled in the procedures. One of their premises is that you must make your own decision about your pregnancy without any outside pressure. They should offer objective and nonjudgmental information and counseling about your available options.

Not every community has a facility that offers abortion services. To find sources of abortion care elsewhere, start with your family doctor or gynecologist. If your doctor is uncomfortable discussing abortion, he or she may be willing to refer you to the nearest physician or clinic that offers counseling and abortion care.

If you are a student, the school nurse or guidance counselor may be able to offer information and support.

At colleges and universities, nursing personnel at the infirmary or the health service are likely to be knowledgeable about pregnancy testing and what options are available. Just how much assistance they provide varies from school to school. State or county health departments, departments of social services, or the Visiting Nurse Association traditionally provide the names of family planning clinics or medical practices that include abortion among their health care services. As mentioned before, however, if a health service receives federal funds, it will not be able to discuss abortion or suggest a referral. In that case, the department of obstetrics and gynecology at most nondenominational hospitals is likely to know nearby clinics that offer skilled abortion services. You can also try the Yellow Pages under "Clinics," "Abortion," or "Family Planning Information Centers."

Note: As mentioned previously, antiabortion groups may advertise in the Yellow Pages and elsewhere as family planning centers or even abortion providers. Their counselors will try to discourage you from terminating your pregnancy. Make certain the clinic you contact actually performs abortions before you make an appointment.

If there are no such clinics in your area, or if existing ones don't provide abortion services, call the nearest Planned Parenthood office. If there isn't one in your community, ask telephone information for the number of the Planned Parenthood office in the urban center nearest to you. Planned Parenthood affiliates offer a broad range of family planning services, including abortion referrals. All their clinics must meet the organization's high standards for care and counseling. Some Planned Parenthood affiliates offer abortions.

Another important resource is the National Abortion Federation. By calling 800-772-9100 toll-free, you can get answers to questions about abortion regulations in your state, the names of the nearest clinics that provide abortion services, and suggestions on where to obtain financial help. (In Washington, D.C., the federation number for abortion information is 202-667-5881.) The federation will give out only the names of its affiliated clinics, which, like Planned Parenthood clinics, maintain certain standards for care and counseling.

Don't delay your search for good-quality abortion services, but don't act in panic either. If it appears that you will have to travel to another community or even to another state to obtain care, be certain that you are pregnant before you make arrangements to travel. Knowing how far the pregnancy has advanced gives you some idea of what procedures you will need—not all clinics offer second-trimester procedures—and this information will help you choose an appropriate clinic.

How to Check Out a Clinic

As with any other facility that offers health care, a clinic or physician providing abortion services should meet certain standards. Before you decide on a particular abortion provider, visit the clinic or doctor and ask questions. Your queries should include the following:

- Do they have a written agreement with a nearby hospital to provide backup emergency care if necessary? How many minutes away by car or ambulance is the hospital? (It should be within a 10- to 20-minute drive, preferably closer.) Do clinic physicians have admitting privileges at that hospital? Does the clinic have the capability of transferring a patient to the hospital?

- Are private spaces set aside for talking with clients? Is printed information available on fees and on the availability of public assistance or other funds? Does the material on fees itemize the services included in the basic fee, and does it list the additional services that might be needed and their costs?
- Is the recovery room supervised at all times by either a licensed nurse or a physician who is on the premises?
- Does the facility have on hand a "crash cart"—the utility cart that holds the equipment for providing cardiac and pulmonary resuscitation? Is at least one staff person on each shift trained in cardiopulmonary resuscitation (CPR)?
- Are drugs on hand to treat cardiac arrest, an asthma attack, an allergic reaction, a seizure, or shock?
- Is the operating room large enough to hold several people as well as the equipment? Is it well lighted?
- Is there an adequate supply of intravenous solutions and at least six units of plasma volume expander available for emergency use? The expander is used as a blood substitute to maintain blood pressure in case of hemorrhage.
- Is there a sterilizing facility for the instruments?
- Does the clinic routinely send all aborted tissue to a pathology laboratory to confirm that pregnancy tissue was indeed removed? (A positive result means the pregnancy was in the uterus and is not an ectopic pregnancy still growing in a fallopian tube or some other place outside the uterus.)
- If this is a second-trimester abortion, is diagnostic ultrasound available? An examination by ultrasound is recommended before *any* second-trimester pregnancy is terminated. After the fourteenth week, the National Abortion Federation requires that its member clinics perform an ultrasound examination for an exact determination of fetal size and position. Some states also may require this of abortion facilities.

With the advent of vacuum aspiration equipment, there is no need today for surgeons to perform first-trimester abortions with a sharp curette, and few do. Because some physicians may still use this method, however, it is a worthwhile precaution to ask the physician what method he or she uses. With a suction curette, pain and bleeding are reduced and the risk of leaving pregnancy tissue behind is decreased.

What Happens at the Clinic

Although the preabortion procedure varies from clinic to clinic or surgeon to surgeon, in general it should cover the same points. A medical assistant or counselor will answer your questions and help you determine whether you need more information or help in arriving at a decision. He or she will want to make certain that you have considered all your options and are comfortable with your decision. Together you will go over the rather lengthy informed consent document you must sign before the abortion can take place. The counselor should be able to answer all questions about the clinic's emergency preparations and facilities and about the actual procedure itself. *As most counselors will tell you, at any point before the abortion actually gets under way, you can change your mind.*

The counselor or a medical assistant will take your medical history. You will be asked about any allergies to local anesthetics, antibiotics, analgesics such as aspirin, and other drugs. You also will be asked about current illnesses or conditions that might affect the performance of the abortion, plus the chance that you might have been exposed to a sexually transmitted disease, including AIDS.

If you have decided to have an abortion, an appointment will be made for the procedure, and several tests will be performed, including the following:

- Either a blood or urine pregnancy test.
- A blood count to check for anemia.
- A blood test to determine if you are Rh negative. If you

are, you will be given Rh immune globulin after the abortion to avoid the risk of Rh sensitization, which could have an adverse effect on any subsequent pregnancy, causing the baby to be born with severe anemia and jaundice. This procedure is also done if the pregnancy is carried to term.

- If there is any possibility you've been exposed to gonorrhea, syphilis, chlamydia, or the AIDS virus, clinic rules may require that you be tested for these diseases. If you have an active STD, the clinic is likely to treat the disease before scheduling your abortion, so the operation does not spread it to the upper part of your reproductive system. In addition, some clinics test for sickle-cell disease and cancers of the reproductive organs.

If you are allergic to the lidocaine family of local anesthetics, general anesthesia may be advised. General anesthesia might also be advisable if you have any condition that makes it difficult for you to be calm and cooperative when surgery is performed with a local anesthetic. If you have any medical condition that might increase the risk of complications during the procedure, the clinic may suggest that a hospital is a better place for having the abortion. Such a complication might be a bleeding disorder, asthma, heart disease, diabetes, or epilepsy that is not well controlled.

Before the Abortion

At most clinics you will receive instructions about what to do to prepare for the abortion. You will be given a urine pregnancy test, a blood test for Rh factor and anemia, and a brief physical examination. If the clinic uses osmotic dilators to dilate the cervix, these often are inserted the day before. If you are having a local anesthetic, you will be advised to eat a very light breakfast or none at all. (If you are having general anesthesia, it is important not to eat or drink for at least eight hours before the surgery, to avoid the chance of vomiting and inhaling food or liquid into your lungs.) Take a shower or bath just before you leave for the clinic and thoroughly wash your genital area. Arrange to have someone who is in your confidence go with you to the clinic in order to provide emotional support and to take you home. If a car isn't available, take a taxi home.

At the clinic, the physician who is going to perform the procedure will conduct a brief physical examination, including checking the size and position of the uterus to determine once again the size and age of the pregnancy. As noted earlier, if the pregnancy is over 14 weeks, many clinics perform an ultrasound examination to ascertain the size of the fetus more accurately. Some clinics perform ultrasound whenever the pregnancy is thought to be 12 weeks or more.

ABORTION PROCEDURES

First-Trimester Vacuum Aspiration

The first trimester of a pregnancy is the first three months—or 13 weeks—counting from the first day of the last normal menstrual period. The most commonly used method of abortion during this period is the vacuum aspiration method, also called vacuum curettage or suction curettage. Vacuum aspiration safely and effectively empties the uterus through the cervical opening.

Although occasionally there are medical or psychological reasons to use general anesthesia, a vacuum abortion most often is carried out with local anesthesia. Moreover, it can be done in various outpatient settings: clinics, private physicians' offices, surgicenters, or, when necessary, hospitals.

For procedures later in the trimester, the cervix must be dilated approximately half an inch in diameter in order to insert the cannula, or vacuum tube. For some abortions, dilators are placed in the cervical canal beforehand to cause it to dilate. Osmotic dilators are short and slender and are made of an absorbent synthetic material. As they absorb moisture, they gradually expand, gently forcing open the cervical os. They are inserted while you lie in the usual position for a pelvic examination. Because some cramping can occur during the insertion, a local anesthetic may be used. Even without anesthesia, some women feel no discomfort, and others have mild cramps. In the unlikely event that severe pain or heavy bleeding occurs later, after the dilators have been inserted, call the clinic or the physician who will be performing the abortion.

At the time of the abortion itself, the physician performs a pelvic exam to determine the size and position of the uterus. A speculum is inserted and the cervix is disinfected. The nearby pain-carrying nerves are numbed with injections of a local anesthetic. Because the cervix has widely spaced nerve receptors, you may not feel the needle, although the injection can set off a wave of cramps. The first injection is made where the tenaculum, a clamplike instrument, will be placed. It holds the cervix during surgical procedures.

After the anesthetic has taken effect, the physician gently straightens the cervix and, if necessary, dilates it further with metal rods in graduated sizes until the os is open enough to accept the cannula. The duration of the pregnancy determines the size of the cannula—as pregnancies develop, the procedure requires a larger cannula. The cannula is connected to an electric vacuum pump, somewhat similar to those used by dentists for aspirating saliva from the mouth. If the pregnancy is less than nine weeks, some clinics use a large syringe to provide the suction.

During vacuum aspiration, the tube is moved around inside the uterus to loosen and remove the pregnancy sac and the thickened lining of the uterus. This procedure takes a few minutes; more advanced pregnancies require more operating time. The vacuum tube is then removed, and the interior of the uterus is explored or "swept" with a curette, a loop-shaped instrument with sharp edges, to make certain all the tissue has been removed. The entire process requires about 10 to 15 minutes from beginning to end, with the actual "vacuuming" taking three to five minutes.

Any discomfort and pain caused by the vacuum procedure varies. Some women feel almost nothing; others find it quite uncomfortable. Toward the end, when most of the tissue has been removed, the uterus contracts. The contraction causes cramps that can range from mild to severe. Fortunately, they seldom last for more than an hour and can be relieved by medication. Most women feel well enough to walk out of the procedure room. Besides the cramping, it is not unusual to have some vaginal bleeding and nausea afterward; nevertheless, most women feel ready to go home within an hour or so.

Second-Trimester Dilation and Evacuation

The second trimester is the second three-month period of a pregnancy—between 14 and 26 weeks of gestation. About 10 percent of abortions in the United States are carried out in the second trimester, chiefly in the first weeks. The most commonly used procedure at this stage is a variation of the curettage method called dilation and evacuation, or D&E. The cervix must be dilated to a greater degree—to more than a half inch—because the pregnancy is more advanced and the fetus is larger. Dilating the cervix may require more time, and the abortion itself takes longer. This technique is preferred for pregnancies that are between 13 and 16 weeks, and very skilled physicians may use it for pregnancies of up to 20 weeks and beyond as well. It is safer than the alternative, an instillation abortion. Like vacuum aspiration, a D&E can be performed in outpatient settings, as long as there is hospital backup available. When it is carried out later in the trimester, it is often done in a hospital.

Undergoing a dilation and evacuation is much like having a vacuum aspiration, although with an increased risk of complications. If local anesthesia is used, the amount of discomfort and the sensations are very similar, and the recovery time is about the same. If general anesthesia is used, there is no pain or discomfort, but the recovery time is usually longer. As in a vacuum aspiration, osmotic dilators are used to open the cervical canal and are inserted beforehand, during a separate clinic visit. At the time of the procedure, after the anesthetic has taken effect, the dilators are removed and, if necessary, the cervical canal is expanded further with metal dilators.

In a D&E, a larger cannula is necessary. It is used in combination with forceps and other instruments that break up the tissue and remove any parts that cannot be suctioned through the tube. To minimize the blood loss that can occur, surgeons frequently use intravenous drugs to encourage the uterus to contract toward the end of the surgery. A D&E takes 20 to 30 minutes. It is the safest method for ending a second-trimester pregnancy and is used for the majority of these advanced pregnancies.

Seldom-Used Methods

Instillation Abortion. A long, hollow needle is inserted through the abdominal wall and into the liquid-filled amniotic sac that surrounds the fetus. A solution of salt, prostaglandin hormones, or urea is slowly instilled through the needle into the amniotic sac. These agents can be used alone or together to induce premature labor and the expulsion of the fetus and placenta. Until the 1970s, instillation abortion was commonly used for terminating second-trimester pregnancies. It has largely been replaced by the safer and much shorter D&E procedure.

An instillation abortion is almost always done in a hospital and may require one or two days of hospitalization. Osmotic dilators are sometimes inserted beforehand to open the cervix. A local anesthetic is preferred because the woman needs to be awake in order to report any unusual sensations that might indicate a reaction to the instillation solution being used. After the injection, there is usually a wait of several hours or more before labor starts, followed by the eventual expulsion of the fetus and placenta. Labor following instillation can be long and painful, and the woman may require generous amounts of pain medication.

If the placenta is not expelled completely during contractions, the physician will try to remove it. If not all of it can be removed, a dilation and curettage (D&C) may be necessary. After the fetus and placenta are expelled, pain and discomfort usually begin to subside. After an hour or two of rest, many women feel well enough to shower. Most hospitals require that women who have had this procedure remain for at least three or four hours after the abortion for observation.

Hysterotomy. Hysterotomy is a major surgical procedure, somewhat like a mini–cesarean section, that requires general or epidural anesthesia and has a higher complication rate (and thus a higher mortality rate) than the other abortion methods. Moreover, any future pregnancies carried to term will almost always require a cesarean delivery because a hysterotomy incision weakens the uterine muscle. Unlike a true cesarean section, the incision is made in the upper part of the uterus, where it is more likely to rupture during the stress of labor. Hysterotomies were used for second-trimester abortions during the brief period right after abortions were made legal everywhere in the United States and before other methods became readily available. Today they are limited to extremely rare second-trimester cases in which a woman has a serious malformation of the uterus, making it dangerous to use the D&E procedure.

Hysterectomy. Hysterectomy, the removal of the uterus itself, is a major operation requiring epidural or general anesthesia. It carries a substantial risk of complications and, consequently, a higher risk of death. Today this surgical procedure is also considered inappropriate as an abortion method and should be performed only when no other method or procedure is possible.

Menstrual Extraction. Not strictly an abortion method, menstrual extraction uses vacuum aspiration to remove the contents of the uterus when a woman believes she may be pregnant, such as after a missed menstrual period or rape, without waiting for a test to confirm pregnancy. Menstrual extraction was used before blood tests that detect a pregnancy as early as eight days after conception became available. With an early pregnancy test readily accessible, the need for menstrual extraction without pregnancy confirmation no longer exists. It is seldom performed.

Abortion Methods Using Drugs

Prostaglandins. Prostaglandins are substances produced naturally by the body. They cause the uterus to contract, among other reactions. Two types of synthetic prostaglandin are used: a vaginal suppository and an injection. They were approved by the FDA in 1977 for the termination of pregnancy between 12 and 24 weeks. They are used in about 1 percent of cases. Usually pregnancies between 13 and 16 weeks can be terminated more easily and with fewer side effects by a D&E. But if a physician is not thoroughly experienced in the D&E technique, prostaglandin suppositories are a safer alternative because they require no surgical expertise. However, a D&E must be done if the prostaglandin procedure fails, as it does in about 5 percent of cases. So a physician who does not do D&Es must be prepared to transfer his patient to a physician who does.

If a suppository is used, the tablet is placed high in the vagina, and the hormone is absorbed by the blood supply in the vaginal walls. Prostaglandins stimulate intense, often painful contractions of the uterus. Compared with injections, suppositories have the advantage of being easy to remove if a severe adverse reaction develops.

The dose of prostaglandin in each tablet needs to be high, and a new tablet has to be inserted every few hours. The constant high dose frequently produces such side effects as extreme nausea, vomiting, and diarrhea. Such reactions, however, often can be alleviated by medications prescribed by the physician. About one-half of the women who abort this way also exhibit a marked rise in temperature. An abortion by means of prostaglandin suppositories takes an average of 14 hours from the insertion of the first tablet to the expulsion of the fetus.

A prostaglandin can also be administered intravenously or as an injection every one to three hours to induce labor contractions. It has many side effects and is not always effective. Like the prostaglandin suppository, it also causes vomiting and diarrhea, but it does not cause a fever. A substantial number of women receiving prostaglandins in any form require a D&C afterward to remove placental tissue that was not expelled. This can occur 10 to 15 percent of the time.

RU 486. A new drug used for termination of early pregnancy, RU 486 blocks the action of progesterone and the maintenance of the implanted embryo. It is administered as a two-step treatment that includes a small dose of prostaglandin and is given only under medical supervision. RU 486, also known as mifepristone (its generic name) and Mifegyne (its trade name), is in use in France, where it was developed, as well as in Great Britain and China. Although this abortion technique is expected to be licensed soon for use in several other countries, at this time it is not available in the United States except for nonabortion research purposes.

An abortion using this drug combination must be done early in a pregnancy. It is considered effective if used within 63 days from the first day of the last menstrual period, or when a woman's period is about five weeks overdue. The drug is given in the form of three tablets taken at one time in the clinic. The woman returns 36 to 48 hours later for either an injection or a vaginal suppository or for pills containing a small dose of prostaglandin.

After receiving the prostaglandin, the woman must remain in the clinic for four hours, during which time most women abort. Prostaglandin side effects can include abdominal pain, diarrhea, nausea, and vomiting, occasionally severe enough to require medication. Afterward, bleeding can last anywhere from one to 35 days, with an average duration of about eight days. If the bleeding is severe, it requires medical intervention. A follow-up visit two weeks later is necessary to ascertain whether the abortion was successful, as it is in 96 percent of cases. For some women, vacuum aspiration or a D&C is required because not all the placental tissue was expelled or, occasionally, because of excessive bleeding or because abortion did not occur.

In France this abortion method requires four visits. One visit is a result of French abortion law and one is for follow-up, as in all abortion procedures. This is one visit more than is required for a surgical abortion, and scientists are hoping to produce a one-time treatment that will reduce the number of visits.

This approach to a medical abortion has the advantage of avoiding complications that result from surgery and anesthesia, putting the procedure more within the woman's control. Many women feel more comfortable with the medical method, compared with the surgical procedure. However, surgical abortions take much less time.

Although most prostaglandin side effects are not serious, one of the prostaglandins used in France, sulprostone, has been blamed for one death and two serious cardiovascular incidents. Because the death involved a heavy smoker, the RU 486 procedure now is not recommended for women who smoke more than 10 cigarettes a day. As an additional safeguard, the French no longer recommend the use of RU 486 for women over 35 or for women who have risk factors for cardiovascular disease.

The publicity surrounding the use of RU 486 as an abortifacient has obscured the fact that this drug also may have other important medical uses. It shows some promise as a way to open the cervix to ease a difficult labor, perhaps reducing the number of cesarean sections. It may prove to be an effective treatment for some breast cancers as well as for benign brain tumors called meningiomas. Other possible uses for RU 486 include the treatment of endometriosis and Cushing's syndrome, a life-threatening disorder of the pituitary gland.

Afterward

If you have had an outpatient procedure, you should not be discharged until you have recovered satisfactorily. While you are in the recovery room, the attending nurse or physician should check your pulse, blood pressure, amount of vaginal bleeding, and general physical condition. If a general anesthesia has been used, you should be fully alert before you are discharged. Before you leave, make an appointment for a follow-up examination. Also get an emergency telephone number in case a complication develops after hours.

You may feel like returning to your usual level of activity immediately or you might want to take it easy. Generally speaking, avoid strenuous exercise for at least a few days. Showering immediately after the abortion is all right, but do not take a bath for several days afterward to avoid the risk of introducing bacteria into the uterus.

Expect some cramps and vaginal bleeding during the following weeks. If the bleeding is heavy—if you are soaking more than one sanitary pad an hour and/or passing clots larger than a half dollar—and it lasts for more than one or two days, call the clinic or physician who performed the abortion. It's normal for light bleeding or spotting or just brownish discharge to occur off and on for as long as a month.

The cramps that usually follow an abortion almost always respond to over-the-counter pain relievers. A nonaspirin product is a better choice because it does not interfere with

---

DANGER SIGNS AFTER ABORTION

Immediately contact your surgeon or the clinic where you received your abortion, or go to the nearest hospital emergency room, if you experience these symptoms:

- a temperature over 100.4° F.
- chills, fatigue, or overall aching feeling
- cramps or abdominal pain that steadily worsens
- an abdomen that feels tender or painful when touched or when you cough, sneeze, walk, or jump
- bleeding that lasts more than three weeks, or bleeding that for three days is more than your usual heaviest menstrual flow
- unusual or bad-smelling vaginal discharge
- pregnancy signs that do not disappear

blood clotting. The standard dose of two tablets every three or four hours usually provides relief. If your cramps are so severe that this regimen does not help, or if the pain becomes steadily worse, call your clinic or doctor.

The drug methergine may be prescribed during the first 24 to 48 hours after the abortion to encourage firm uterine contractions and limit the amount of bleeding. If this causes severe cramps or pain that spreads downward to your thighs, call your practitioner. It may be necessary to stop taking the drug to ease the cramps.

Because infection is possible after an abortion, take your temperature if you have chills or feel feverish. If you are taking aspirin or a similar analgesic, take your temperature *before* you take the pills. (They lower body temperature.) If you have a temperature over 100.4° F, call your physician.

Do not use tampons (use sanitary pads), douche, or have intercourse for two weeks after the abortion. If you have had a later abortion, you may develop breast milk. To stop it, wear a snug-fitting bra day and night for two or three days. Avoid any stimulation of the nipples and don't squeeze the milk from your breasts, since this increases milk production.

Contraception After Abortion

You need to start using a contraceptive method before you begin having intercourse again. Most likely, your surgeon or the clinic counselor will discuss contraception with you; if not, raise the question yourself. If your pregnancy was the result of a contraceptive failure, you may want to change methods.

If your abortion takes place before the end of the tenth week of pregnancy, before the uterus becomes large and soft, it is possible to be sterilized when you have the abortion. However, it is only in large urban centers that you may find a clinic able to provide abortion and sterilization services simultaneously. (Such clinics are able to do both procedures at once because they use local anesthesia for both.) Most of the time surgeons who perform sterilizations prefer to use general anesthesia, which requires hospitalization and is more expensive.

EFFECTIVENESS

Early abortions by whatever techniques have low failure rates. Pregnancies continue in only 0.1 to 0.3 percent of abortions. Incomplete abortions that require a follow-up procedure occur in a very small percentage of women.

COMPLICATIONS

In 1965, before the general availability of legal abortion services, abortions accounted for nearly 17 percent of all deaths due to childbirth and pregnancy. Today, death from abortion is rare. Between 1972 and 1982, the following mortality rates were recorded: vacuum procedure, one death per 125,000 procedures; dilation and evacuation, one death per 20,000; instillation procedure, one death per 10,000; hysterotomy and hysterectomy, one death in 223 procedures. First-trimester abortions are the safest. Indeed, the risk of death for all abortions is about one-eighth that of giving birth to a child. In the second trimester the mortality rates for abortion and childbirth are the same, eight deaths per 100,000.

Hemorrhage

The most common complication immediately after an abortion is excessive bleeding. Of every 1,000 women who have abortions, between two and 10 have excessive bleeding. A very small proportion bleed so severely they need a blood transfusion. Hemorrhage occurs when the uterus is not completely cleared of pregnancy tissue or when it does not contract enough after the abortion has been completed. It can also occur if the tissues of the uterus, cervix, or vagina have been injured. Heavy bleeding is usually prevented by using a drug to encourage the uterus to contract (the contraction of the uterus closes the blood vessels) and by using a local rather than a general anesthetic. General anesthesia appears to reduce the strength of uterine contractions and is associated with greater blood loss. Massaging the uterus also encourages contractions. Making sure all the placenta has been expelled or removed from the uterus helps to prevent blood loss. It is especially important that this procedure be done thoroughly in a second-trimester procedure, where the uterus is bigger and tissue is more apt to be overlooked.

If you have a bleeding disorder or are taking medication that slows blood clotting, you are at a greater risk of hemorrhage. If you regularly take aspirin, you may also be at risk for prolonged bleeding.

Incomplete Abortion

An abortion is not complete if any fetal or placental tissue remains in the uterus. Most obvious indications of an unfinished abortion are cramps and bleeding. If you continue to experience the usual signs of pregnancy—nausea, breast soreness, and fatigue—seek treatment.

In some instances of incomplete abortion, however, you may have no signs of pregnancy or any other indication that the abortion was not thoroughly done. For this reason it is important to see your surgeon for a postabortion examination, which is usually scheduled at the time of the abortion. If it is difficult to return to the clinic where you had the abortion, have this checkup performed by your local physician or health care provider.

Infection

Cramps, pain that gets worse, fever, a vaginal discharge, pelvic discomfort, and feeling unwell may be signs of an infection in the uterus or fallopian tubes. The presence of tissue fragments in the uterus may increase the risk of infection.

If you suspect an infection, seek medical care at once. Most infections respond well to antibiotics if they are caught early. An infection that becomes severe can require hospitalization and vigorous treatment with intravenous antibiotics. An infection of the uterus and fallopian tubes can cause scar tissue and adhesions to develop, making it difficult or impossible to become pregnant at some future time. Severe infections can necessitate a hysterectomy and the loss of the uterus, fallopian tubes, and ovaries.

To avoid the chance of infection, many clinics routinely provide prophylactic antibiotics. For most women tetracycline or a similar antibiotic is given just before the abortion, or immediately afterward, and continued for one or two days. Women at risk for pelvic inflammatory disease may be given a somewhat longer antibiotic regimen. In addition, prophylactic antibiotics are often prescribed for the woman who has an artificial heart valve, a heart valve disorder, or another congenital heart abnormality. If you have one of these problems, discuss the use of antibiotics with your heart specialist and the surgeon performing the abortion.

Injuries to the Uterus, Cervix, or Nearby Organs

Cervical lacerations, or tears, can occur when tissue is forced through a cervical canal that has not been sufficiently dilated. Such lacerations occur more frequently in a woman who has never been pregnant before and has a small, rigid cervix. A cervical tear may need suturing to stop the bleeding. Such injuries are much less likely to occur if laminaria are used beforehand to dilate the cervix. The physician's skill in holding the cervix with the tenaculum is an important factor in avoiding cervical injury.

The uterus can be perforated by one of the instruments used during the procedure. In severe perforations, the instrument goes through the wall of the uterus and damages the uterine ligaments on either side or enters the abdominal cavity. Simple puncture wounds are likely to close up and heal by themselves, but if nearby organs have been injured, emergency surgery may be necessary. If a blood vessel has been damaged, it will have to be sutured shut. If blood loss is not extensive, the abortion can be completed, perhaps with a laparoscopic examination to determine the extent of the trauma (see Chapter 11). Severe blood loss is best dealt with in a hospital. Exploratory surgery or laparoscopy may be required, and a transfusion may be needed.

Drug Reactions and Other Adverse Effects

A reaction can be caused by one of the local anesthetics, which are similar to Novocain; the antibiotics tetracycline, ampicillin, or amoxicillin; and the drugs methergine or oxytocin, which may be used for stimulating contractions.

As noted earlier, if prostaglandins are used in abortions, they can cause the unpleasant side effects of vomiting, nausea, and diarrhea. Many doctors routinely prescribe medication to treat these reactions.

In an instillation abortion, the saline solution can be injected into a blood vessel, causing death. Also, a blood vessel or the uterus can be damaged by the needle. If saline is mistakenly injected into a muscle, it may destroy the tissue in the immediate area.

Long-Term Complications

Early first-trimester abortions that are carried out with the suction technique appear to have no negative effects on future reproductive health. Vacuum aspiration abortions do not increase the frequency of spontaneous abortions (miscarriages), premature deliveries, or low-birth-weight babies. Fertility is not affected by any abortion that is carefully performed, especially when the abortion is done early in a pregnancy. A postabortion complication, however, especially an infection, can increase the risk of infertility. Injuries to the cervix incurred during abortions (or during childbirth) may increase the chance of developing cervical problems during a subsequent pregnancy. Such an injury may cause the cervical canal gradually to widen and open because of the pressure of the growing fetus, until the woman aborts spontaneously. Generally this problem can be treated successfully by temporarily tying the cervix shut until labor begins or the pregnancy has reached its full term.

Cost

First-trimester abortions done on an outpatient basis in a free-standing clinic generally cost between $200 and $350. Because second-trimester procedures are somewhat more complicated, they cost between $350 and $450 if carried out between the thirteenth and sixteenth weeks. After the sixteenth week, the cost rises approximately $100 per week. An abortion late in the second trimester can cost more than $1,000. Fees have increased only slightly since abortion was made legal in all states in 1973, but any legislative changes that affect the financial support of abortion services may force some clinics to increase their charges.

Some health insurance plans cover the cost of induced abortions for employees or their dependents. Others pay only for abortions necessary for medical reasons. Health Maintenance Organizations (HMOs) in general are likely to include all induced abortions in their coverage; Blue Cross and Blue Shield may include only medically necessary abortions. Whether your health insurance coverage includes this procedure depends on the company writing the insurance or on your individual plan. Many health insurance plans include abortion under maternity benefits.

If you don't know what your health plan coverage includes, ask your company's personnel office or the benefits office for a copy of your benefits sheet, or call the insurance company directly. It is easier to remain anonymous by talking to the insurance company. You will need to know your benefits identification number or the name of your health benefits package (such as "Master Medical") when requesting information.

Employees of the U.S. government, including those in the armed services, are not covered for abortion services. Similarly, women who work for state or city governments also may not be covered for abortion by their health insurance.

If you don't have health coverage and can't afford to pay for an abortion, there may be other sources of funds available in your community. Women's health groups or feminist groups may make loans or outright grants of money. State or local chapters of the National Abortion Rights Action League (NARAL) and the National Organization for Women (NOW) may have a fund earmarked for women who need abortion services. If you can't find these organizations in your local telephone directory, call their Washington headquarters. The number for NARAL is 202-408-4600; for NOW, it is 202-331-0066. Planned Parenthood affiliates also may have access to similar funds, such as the Justice Fund. The National Abortion Federation (800-772-9100) also has information on sources of financial assistance.

Counselors at abortion clinics should be knowledgeable about the resources available in their community. Some cities may have little-known private foundations that help women pay for abortions. If you need financial help, pursue the available resources early and vigorously.

17

Breast-feeding and Contraception

Your birth control needs often change after you have a child. You may now feel your family is complete, or you may want to postpone your next pregnancy. If you are nursing, you need to know what contraceptive choices are appropriate during this period and what effect some contraceptives might have on the quality or quantity of breast milk.

CONTRACEPTIVE EFFECT OF BREAST-FEEDING

Breast-feeding, or lactation, delays the return to ovulation. This situation leads to amenorrhea, or lack of menstruation, which lasts a variable length of time after the birth of a child and is known as lactational amenorrhea. The length of the delay depends a great deal on how completely you nurse your baby. Frequent, around-the-clock nursing appears to prevent the secretion of hormones necessary for an egg to mature in the ovaries. Associated with this state of infertility are high levels of prolactin in your body. Prolactin is necessary for the production of a milk supply, and its secretion depends on the frequency and duration of the baby's suckling. The more a baby nurses, the higher your prolactin levels become and the less chance you have of ovulating.

Lactational amenorrhea appears to be a very effective contraceptive. During the first six months after childbirth, *women who exclusively breast-feed their infants and have not begun to menstruate again* have less than a 2 percent risk of pregnancy. The risk of pregnancy increases if menstruation resumes. This is more likely as time passes, or if you supplement breast-feeding with other foods. Adequate protection from pregnancy may last substantially longer than six months for many breast-feeding women.

The majority of breast-feeding women in the United States give their infants solid foods or bottle milk early in life, and this practice leads to the early return of ovulation. If you begin supplementary feedings, the reduction in suckling allows your body to ovulate. Obviously, for the new mother who is not breast-feeding or is only partially breast-feeding, the period of amenorrhea and nonovulation after childbirth can be brief. Once amenorrhea ends, as is demonstrated by

---

WHAT IS EXCLUSIVE BREAST-FEEDING?

There is a strong positive correlation between the frequency and duration of suckling and lack of ovulation. If you wish to use breast-feeding as a means of contraception, you must be exclusively or almost exclusively nursing, which is

- nursing frequently, whenever the baby is hungry, both day and night
- not offering the infant a bottle, pacifier, or other artificial nipple
- not supplementing breast milk regularly with milk or other sources of calories

When any of these criteria is *not* met, you are no longer exclusively or almost breast-feeding. You should begin to use an additional method of contraception if menstruation resumes or if you are no longer breast-feeding.

any vaginal bleeding after the first month postpartum, a contraceptive is necessary to protect against pregnancy. Many women choose to use some contraceptive protection even before the first vaginal bleeding in order to avoid even the small risk that a fertile first ovulation might precede any evidence of bleeding.

It is a good idea to begin thinking about postpartum contraceptive methods before you have your baby. Since many couples resume sexual intercourse within the first weeks after childbirth, nonnursing and partially nursing women should begin to use a contraceptive immediately. Fully nursing women may not need a contraceptive as soon, but many begin to use barrier methods after the six-week postpartum checkup.

CONTRACEPTIVE METHODS FOR THE BREAST-FEEDING WOMAN

Although some women return to the birth control methods they had been using before they became pregnant, for many others, childbirth and breast-feeding lead to a different approach to contraception. Most available birth control methods can be used safely by the woman who has just given birth or is breast-feeding. Some are better than others.

Condoms pose no risk to either mother or child and offer protection against STDs and AIDS. Because a nursing mother's vagina is less naturally lubricated than normal, the use of a lubricated condom, or a condom plus a spermicide or a nonoily lubricant, can make this method of contraception comfortable and appealing.

Whether or not you are breast-feeding, it is necessary to wait until postpartum involution of the uterus has occurred (when the uterus shrinks back to normal size and its normal place, and the cervix is closed, after about six weeks) before being fitted for a *diaphragm or cervical cap.* If you have used one of these methods previously, you need to be refitted at this time, because the shape and size of the cervix and upper vagina may have changed with childbirth.

Spermicides have not been shown to have an effect on breast-feeding, even though extremely small amounts may be absorbed into the maternal blood. Since vaginal dryness is common during lactation, some women may find that spermicides, either used alone or with a barrier method, make intercourse more comfortable.

The sponge is available in only one size, so it often does not fit the vagina snugly after childbirth. As a result, the contraceptive sponge has had a high failure rate in women who have had children.

Intrauterine devices (IUDs) are well suited to nursing women because they are convenient and effective. Neither the progesterone released from the Progestasert nor the copper of the ParaGard appear to have any effect on breast-feeding or on the infant. The risk of expulsion can be reduced if the IUD is inserted when the uterus has returned to normal size, at approximately six weeks postpartum. Recent evidence suggests that the chance of discomfort is reduced when the insertion is performed during lactation.

Vasectomy is an excellent method if no more children are wanted, because it is almost always permanent. Counseling is particularly important if a couple is making this decision shortly before or after the birth of a child.

If a *tubal occlusion* is performed, general anesthesia can pass into the breast milk and may have effects that can be disruptive to breast-feeding. Therefore, a local anesthetic is frequently recommended if this procedure is performed at this time. Both general anesthesia and heavy sedation have been associated with less milk production for as long as two weeks afterward and with problems in beginning successful breast-feeding. They appear to interfere with the establishment of a good sucking response. Moreover, if a tubal occlusion separates you from your baby for more than a few hours, it may disrupt the psychological bonding process and also the development of an adequate milk supply. Because this is a permanent method, counseling is important beforehand.

The *minipill* and *Norplant* are not the methods of first choice for the lactating woman. Although small amounts of the hormone pass into the milk, there is no current evidence of adverse effects on the infant. Generally, though, it is wiser to avoid this early exposure to hormones. If you do choose the minipill and it's at all feasible, take the pill at the beginning of the longest interval between feedings, to minimize the amount of hormone reaching the baby. But do so only if this timing is consistent with providing good contraceptive protection (see Chapter 8).

Combined oral contraceptives are not recommended for the breast-feeding woman. The estrogen in these pills decreases, the milk supply. This decrease, in turn, leads to the earlier use of supplemental feeding and an early end to breast-feeding. If combined pills must be used, avoid them until lactation has been well established. As with the progestin-only pill, take the combined pill at the beginning of the longest interval between feedings to minimize the hormonal dose received by the baby, and try to provide extra breast-feeding to maintain the milk supply.

Fertility awareness methods generally are not useful after childbirth and during breast-feeding. Basal body temperature patterns are erratic and cannot be used to predict ovulation. Cervical mucus patterns also vary, and changes are harder to detect.

In general, barrier methods are the best complements to breast-feeding, because they have no effect on the infant and their effectiveness is enhanced by the contraceptive effect of nursing.

18

New Contraceptive Options

Over the years, a number of new methods of birth control have been described as likely to become available in the near future. Most of these still have not made it to the marketplace. Since the Pill and the IUD were introduced more than 30 years ago, the only new methods to appear have been the contraceptive sponge, contraceptive film, and Norplant. We describe here four contraceptives that, at this time, seem the most likely to become available in the United States during the 1990s.

FEMALE CONDOMS

Two types of condoms for women are in the last stages of being readied for marketing. Both offer extra protection against sexually transmitted diseases as well as prevent pregnancy.

The *Reality Vaginal Pouch* is a soft, loose-fitting sheath with a flexible polyurethane ring at each end. The ring inside the closed end is used to insert the sheath into the vagina and to hold the closed end near the cervix. Although it is positioned much like a diaphragm, it does not have to fit quite as well. The second ring forms the open end of the sheath and remains outside the vagina, where it covers the labia. The Reality Pouch has several advantages over a male condom: It can be put in place before intercourse begins; a partially erect penis can slip into it; and the penis does not have to be removed from the vagina while still erect. The polyurethane material of the pouch is stronger than latex, is not damaged by the use of oils, and reportedly does not significantly decrease sensation. Like male condoms, the Reality Pouch is used only once.

The *Bikini Condom* is made of latex and is held in place with thin latex straps that fit the body much like a bikini. It covers the genital area and holds a rolled-up latex pouch against the vagina. This condom also can be put on before intercourse. Just before penetration, the pouch is pushed slightly into the vagina with the fingers. The penis pushes it the rest of the way. The pouch is approximately twice as thick as the thickest male condom, and both sides are lubricated to make insertion and removal easier. A major disadvantage of the Bikini Condom is that the pouch can be pulled accidentally from the vagina during intercourse or when the penis is withdrawn after intercourse. Moreover, the latex straps occasionally pinch the skin or pull the pubic hair. Worn by men as well as women, the Bikini Condom is used only once.

Tests on the female condom will be completed in 1992; it is expected to be available to the public in 1993.

VAGINAL RINGS

Vaginal rings are devices made of silicone rubber that resemble the rim of a small diaphragm without the dome, about 2 inches in diameter. The ring is placed in the vagina in any position, where the silicone releases a constant, small amount of hormone, which is absorbed by blood vessels in the vaginal walls. Because the hormones are administered so directly, the amount required for adequate contraception is very low. Two types of rings are being developed: (1) a ring that contains estrogen and progestin and is worn continuously for three weeks and then not worn for one week to permit a menstrual period, and (2) another ring that contains only progesterone, the natural hormone, and is intended for use by lactating women. It is left in place continuously.

Either one of these rings can be removed for a short time for cleaning or if the wearer or her partner finds it uncomfortable during intercourse. Some women find it necessary to remove the ring before they have a bowel movement, to prevent the ring from being pushed out. Only one ring size will be sold because a close fit is not necessary. Each type will contain enough hormones for several cycles.

TIMED-RELEASE INJECTABLE MICROSPHERES

A progestin-only injectable contraceptive, currently being clinically tested, contains tiny spheres about the size of sugar grains. The microspheres permit the progestin to be released gradually over a 90-day period, providing a constant level of hormone to the body. The side effects seen in the early clinical studies are those usually associated with progestin-only contraceptives, although there were more instances of heavy or prolonged bleeding and fewer instances of light or absent periods.

DEPO-PROVERA

The long-acting injectable progestin, Depo-Provera, has been available as a contraceptive in other countries since 1978, and it is gradually becoming a contraceptive option in the United States. Depo-Provera has been approved as a contraceptive in 90 countries, and more than 5 million women are using it. In the United States it has been approved as a treatment for several conditions, including some endometrial cancers and endometriosis. When its manufacturer, the Upjohn Company, sought authorization to market Depo-Provera as a contraceptive in the United States, however, the application was rejected by the FDA because studies found some adverse effects in dogs and monkeys given the drug.

However, long-term experience with Depo-Provera has revealed few problems. Five worldwide studies have recorded no complications more serious than those associated with the progestin-only pill—menstrual cycle irregularities, including amenorrhea. For some women, the reduction in menstrual blood flow, cramps, pain, premenstrual symptoms, and midmonth ovulatory pain that this drug may cause is beneficial. Because it contains no estrogen, Depo-Provera can be used by women who are at risk for cardiovascular complications and by women who experienced serious side effects from an oral contraceptive that contained estrogen. Moreover, it has not been seen to increase the risk of thrombophlebitis.

Depo-Provera is taken as an injection every three months. Its protection is effective for four to six weeks beyond the three months, thereby allowing a margin of protection. Another characteristic is that fertility will not return promptly. After discontinuing this method, the return to normal fertility may be delayed for unpredictable lengths of time up to several months. The failure rate of this birth control drug is usually less than one pregnancy per 100 women per year.

In the United States, Depo-Provera is available to treat endometriosis and heavy menstrual periods that cause anemia. It is also used to treat recurring, inoperable endometrial cancers. In the past few years, as its safety as a contraceptive in other countries has become more obvious, an increasing number of U.S. family planning clinics have offered it for birth control. Although the FDA has not approved it for this use, in the United States clinicians may prescribe drugs for purposes other than the original ones for which they were approved.

References

Adler, N. E., H. P. David, et al. "Psychological Responses After Abortion." *Science* 248 (April 6, 1990): 41–44.

Alvarez, F., V. Brache, et al. "New Insights on the Mode of Action of Intrauterine Contraceptive Devices in Women." *Fertility and Sterility* 49, no. 5 (May 1988): 768–73.

American Medical Association. *Encyclopedia of Medicine.* New York: Random House, 1989.

Andrews, W. C., and K. P. Jones. "Therapeutic Uses of Oral Contraceptives." *Dialogues in Contraception* 3, no. 3 (Winter 1991): 1–8. Published by the University of Southern California School of Medicine, Los Angeles.

Antarsh, L. "AVSC Embarks upon a Program to Teach Local Anesthesia for Female Sterilization." *AVSC News* 27, no. 3 (October 1989): 1–2. Published by the Association for Voluntary Surgical Contraception.

Beresford, T. *Unsure About Your Pregnancy?* Washington, D.C.: National Abortion Federation, 1990.

Billings, E., and A. Westmore. *The Billings Method.* New York: Random House, 1980.

Boston Women's Health Book Collective. *The New Our Bodies, Ourselves.* New York: Simon & Schuster, 1984.

Bracken, M. B., K. G. Hellenbrand, and T. R. Holford. "Contraception Delay After Oral Contraceptive Use: The Effect of Estrogen Dose." *Fertility and Sterility* 53, no. 1 (January 1990): 21–27.

"Breastfeeding and Contraception." *Outlook* 8, no. 1 (March 1990): 2–10.

"British Study Suggests Long-Term Pill Use Before First Term Pregnancy Raises Risk of Breast Cancer." *Family Planning Perspectives* 19, no. 6 (November/December 1987): 267–69.

Broome, M., and K. Fotherby. "Clinical Experience with the Progestogen-Only Pill." *Contraception* 42, no. 5 (November 1990): 489–95.

Brown, H. P. "The Pill and Breast Cancer." *Health and Sexuality* 1, no. 1 (Fall 1990): 6–7.

Bullough, V. L., and B. Bullough. *Contraception.* Buffalo: Prometheus Books, 1990.

"Can You Rely on Condoms?" *Consumer Reports,* March 1989, pp. 135–41.

Cancer and Steroid Hormone Study of the Centers for Disease Control and the National Institute of Child Health and Human Development. "Oral-Contraceptive Use and the Risk of Breast Cancer." *New England Journal of Medicine* 315 (August 14, 1986): 405–11.

Cates, W., Jr., A. E. Washington, et al. "The Pill, Chlamydia and PID." *Family Planning Perspectives* 17, no. 4 (July/August 1985): 175–76.

Cherniak, D. *A Book About Birth Control.* Montreal: Montreal Health Press, 1987.

Darney, P. D., E. Atkinson, et al. "Acceptance and Perceptions of Norplant Among Users in San Francisco, USA." *Studies in Family Planning* 21, no. 3 (May/June 1990): 152–60.

Davis, K. "The Story of the Pill." *American Heritage,* August/September 1978: 80–90.

"Depo-medroxyprogesterone Acetate (DMPA) and Cancer: Memorandum from a WHO Meeting." *Bulletin of the World Health Organization* 64, no. 3 (1986): 375–82.

"Diagnostic and Therapeutic Technology Assessment of Intrauterine Devices," ed. H. M. Cole. *Journal of the American Medical Association* 261, no. 14 (April 14, 1989): 2127–30.

"Do Studies Point to Real Breast Cancer Risk with OCs?" *Contraceptive Technology Update,* May 1990, pp. 69–70.

"Does Oral Contraceptive Use Lead to Delayed Contraception?" *Contraceptive Technology Update,* April 1990, pp. 63–64.

"Female Condoms Scheduled to Reach U.S. Market This Year." *Contraceptive Technology Update* 12, no. 8 (August 1991): 117–28.

Fertility Control, ed. S. L. Corson, R. J. Derman, and L. B. Tyrer. Boston: Little, Brown, 1985.

Forrest, J. D. "The End of IUD Marketing in the United States: What Does It Mean for American Women?" *Family Planning Perspectives* 18, no. 2 (March/April 1986): 52–57.

Fotherby, K. "The Progestogen-Only Pill." In *Contraception—Science and Practice,* ed. M. Filshie and J. Guillebaud. London: Butterworths, 1989.

"A Fresh Look at Barrier Contraceptives." *Contemporary OB/GYN,* March 1988, pp. 132–52.

Gallagher, D. M., and G. A. Richwald. *Fitting the Cervical Cap: A Handbook for Clinicians.* Los Gatos, Calif.: Cervical Cap, Ltd., 1989.

"General Anesthesia for Female Sterilization Under Scrutiny." *Contraceptive Technology Update,* February 1990, pp. 28–30.

Gold, R. B. *Abortion and Women's Health: A Turning Point for America?* New York: Alan Guttmacher Institute, 1990.

Goldstein, M. "Vasectomy and Vasectomy Reversal." In *Current Therapy in Endocrinology and Metabolism–3.* Philadelphia: B. C. Decker, 1988.

Goldstein, M., and M. Feldberg. *The Vasectomy Book.* Boston: Houghton Mifflin, 1982.

Grimes, D. A. "Intrauterine Devices and Pelvic Inflammatory Disease: Recent Developments." *Contraception* 36, no. 1 (July 1987): 97–109.

Grimes, D. A. "IUD Insertion: A Clinical Refresher." *The Female Patient* 14, no. 2: 51–54.

Guidelines for Breastfeeding in Family Planning and Child Survival Programs, ed. M. H. Labbok, P. Koniz-Booher, et al. Washington, D.C.: Georgetown University Press, 1990.

Guillebaud, J. *The Pill.* Oxford, England: Oxford University Press, 1980.

Harlap, S., K. Kost, and J. D. Forrest. *Preventing Pregnancy, Protecting Health: A New Look at Birth Control Choices in the United States.* New York: Alan Guttmacher Institute, 1991.

Hatcher, R. A., F. Stewart, J. Trussell, et al. *Contraceptive Technology.* New York: Irvington, 1990.

Having an Abortion? Your Guide to Good Care. Washington, D.C.: National Abortion Federation, 1990.

"The Health Benefits of Oral Contraceptives." *Contraception Report* 1, no. 3: 3–5.

Henshaw, S., and J. Van Vort. "Abortion Services in the United States, 1987 and 1988." *Family Planning Perspectives* 22, no. 3 (May/June 1990): 102–143.

Hilts, P. J. "U.S. Is Decades Behind Europe in Contraceptives, Experts Report." *New York Times*, February 15, 1990.

Himes, N. E. *Medical History of Contraception.* New York: Schocken Books, 1970.

"Is Anti-Abortion Movement Undermining Contraception?" *Contraceptive Technology Update* 12, no. 9 (September 1991): 133–38.

"Is It Safe to Prescribe Oral Contraceptives Until Menopause?" *Contraceptive Technology Update* 10, no. 12 (December 1989): 167–71.

Kaeser, L. "Reconsidering the Age Limits on Pill Use." *Family Planning Perspectives* 21, no. 6 (November/December 1989): 273–74.

Koonin, L., K. D. Kochanek, et al. "Abortion Surveillance, United States, 1988." *Morbidity and Mortality Weekly Report* 40, no. SS-2 (July 1991): 15–42.

"Lack of Data on 'Morning After' Pill Confounds Clinicians." *Contraceptive Technology Update* 8, no. 11 (November 1987): 137–40.

Lee, N., G. Rubin, and R. Borucki. "The Intrauterine Device and Pelvic Inflammatory Disease Revisited: New Results from the Women's Health Study." *Obstetrics and Gynecology* 72, no. 1 (July 1988): 1–6.

Li, S., M. Goldstein, J. Zhu, and D. Huber. "The No-Scalpel Vasectomy." *Journal of Urology* 145 (February 1991): 341–44.

McClure, D. A., and D. A. Edelman. "Worldwide Method Effectiveness of the Today Vaginal Contraceptive Sponge." In *Advances in Contraception.* Lancaster, England: MTP Press, 1985.

McDonald, T. L. *The Cervical Cap Handbook.* Iowa City: Emma Goldman Clinic for Women, 1988.

"Minilaparotomy and Laparoscopy: Safe, Effective, and Widely Used." *Population Reports,* Series C, no. 9 (May 1985). Published by Johns Hopkins University.

"Minipills Remain Choice for 'Specialty Patient' Groups." *Contraceptive Technology Update* 9, no. 2 (February 1988): 13–15.

Mosher, W. D. "Contraceptive Practice in the United States, 1982–1988." *Family Planning Perspectives* 22, no. 5 (September/October 1990): 198–205.

National Research Council and the Institute of Medicine. *Developing New Contraceptives: Obstacles and Opportunities,* ed. L. Mastroianni, Jr., P. J. Donaldson, and T. T. Kane. Washington, D.C.: National Academy Press, 1990.

"Natural Family Planning an Appealing Method for Some." *Contraceptive Technology Update* 11, no. 2 (February 1990): 21–28.

"New Studies Find No Link Between Spermicide Use and Heightened Risk of Congenital Malformations." *Family Planning Perspectives* 20, no. 1 (January/February 1988): 42–43.

"No Increase in Risk of PID for IUD Users Who Are Married or Cohabitating with One Sexual Partner." *Family Planning Perspectives* 21, no. 1 (January/February 1989): 35–36.

"Norplant: 'Most Effective Reversible Method in World.'" *Contraceptive Technology Update* 11, no. 1 (January 1990): 1–8.

Norplant Contraceptive Subdermal Implants: Manual for Clinicians. New York: Population Council, 1990.

North, B. B., and B. W. Vorhauer. "Use of the Today Contraceptive Sponge in the United States." *International Journal of Fertility* 30, no. 1 (1985): 81–84.

"OC Compliance and Contraceptive Failure." *Contraception Report* 1, no. 4: 3–6.

"Oral Contraceptive Association with Breast Cancer Is Not Conclusive, FDA Advisory Committee Agrees; Recent Studies Do Not Support Labeling Change." *FDC Reports* 51, no. 2 (January 9, 1989): 13–14.

"Oral Contraceptives and Breast Cancer." *Health and Sexuality* 1, no. 1 (Fall 1990): 1–5.

Ortiz, M. E., and H. B. Croxatto. "The Mode of Action of IUDs." *Contraception* 36, no. 1 (July 1987): 37–53.

Overmyer, R. H. "In-Office Contraceptive Implant Is Effective, Long-Acting, Reversible." *Modern Medicine* 59 (January 1991).

"Pill Appears to Provide Long-Term Protection Against Endometrial Cancer and Ovarian Cancer." *Family Planning Perspectives* 19, no. 3 (May/June 1987): 126–27.

"Pill Users Face Increased Risk of Cervical Cancer, But Decreased Risk of Other Genital Cancers." *Family Planning Perspectives* 21, no. 1 (January/February 1989): 33.

Pollner, F. "OC Age Limit Is Out of Date, FDA Advisory Panel Decides." *Medical World News*, November 27, 1989, pp. 12–13.

"Postcoital Contraception: A Necessary, Important Option." *Contraceptive Technology Update* 10, no. 11 (November 1989): 145–53.

"Postcoital Contraceptives Available, But Seldom Used." *Contraceptive Technology Update* 10, no. 5 (May 1989): 67–68.

Potts, M. "Birth Control Methods in the United States." *Family Planning Perspectives* 20, no. 6 (November/December 1988): 288–97.

"Progestogens in the Pill Modify Levels of Serum Lipids, WHO Study Finds." *Family Planning Perspectives* 21, no. 3 (May/June 1989): 141–42.

"Protective Effects of Oral Contraceptives Against Ovarian and Endometrial Cancers." *Contraception Report* 1, no. 3: 6–7.

Richwald, G. A., S. Greenland, et al. "Effectiveness of the Cavity-Rim Cervical Cap: Results of a Large Clinical Study." *Obstetrics and Gynecology* 74, no. 2 (August 1989): 143–48.

Schildkraut, J. M., B. S. Hulka, and W. E. Wilkinson. "Oral Contraceptives and Breast Cancer: A Case-Controlled Study with Hospital and Community Controls." *Obstetrics and Gynecology* 76, no. 3, pt. 1 (September 1990): 395–402.

Schlesselman, J. J. "Oral Contraceptives and Breast Cancer." *American Journal of Obstetrics and Gynecology* 163, no. 4, pt. 2 (October 1990): 1379–87.

Shapiro, H. I. *The New Birth Control Book.* New York: Prentice Hall, 1988.

"Should Surgical Sterilization Be Considered Reversible?" *Contraceptive Technology Update,* June 1989.

Silber, S. J. *How Not to Get Pregnant.* New York: Charles Scribner's Sons/Warner Books, 1987.

Silvestre, L., C. Dubois, et al. "Voluntary Interruption of Pregnancy with Mifepristone (RU 486) and a Prostaglandin Analogue." *New England Journal of Medicine* 322, no. 10 (March 8, 1990): 645–48.

Sivin, I. "IUDs Are Contraceptives, Not Abortifacients: A Comment on Research and Belief." *Studies in Family Planning* 20, no. 6 (November/December 1989): 355–59.

Soderstrom, R. "IUDs Now Require Patients' Informed Consent." *Contemporary OB/GYN,* September 15, 1988.

Spark, R. F. *Male Sexual Health.* New York: Consumer Reports Books, 1991.

"Sponge Used More for STD Prevention Than Contraception." *Contraceptive Technology Update* 11, no. 10 (October 1990): 145–60.

Stampfer, M. J., W. C. Willett, et al. "A Prospective Study of Past Use of Oral Contraceptive Agents and Risk of Cardiovascular Diseases." *New England Journal of Medicine* 319, no. 20 (November 17, 1988): 1313–17.

Standards for Abortion Care. Washington, D. C.: National Abortion Federation, 1988.

"Sterilization a Popular, Effective Method of Birth Control." *Contraceptive Technology Update* 11, no. 4 (April 1990): 55–64.

Stewart, F. H., F. J. Guest, et al. *Understanding Your Body.* New York: Bantam, 1987.

Sutherland, R. "Vasectomy to Cut HIV Infectivity May Not Live Up to Billing." *Medical Post*, May 21, 1991, p. 29.

Tatum, H. J., and S. Waldman, "The New ParaGard Copper T 380A Intrauterine Device." *Medical Digest* 9, no. 1 (Winter 1989): 1–5.

Thorogood, M., and M. P. Vessey. "An Epidemiologic Survey of Cardiovascular Disease in Women Taking Oral Contraceptives." *American Journal of Obstetrics and Gynecology* 163, no. 1, pt. 2 (July 1990): 274–81.

Torres, A., and J. D. Forrest. "Why Do Women Have Abortions?" *Family Planning Perspectives* 20, no. 4 (July/August 1988): 169–76.

Trussell, J., and K. Kost. "Contraceptive Failure in the United States: A Critical Review of the Literature." *Studies in Family Planning* 18, no. 5 (September/October 1987): 237–83.

Trussell, J., R. A. Hatcher, et al. "Contraceptive Failure in the United States: An Update." *Studies in Family Planning* 21, no. 1 (January/February 1990): 51–54.

U. S. Congress, Office of Technology Assessment. *Infertility: Medical and Social Choices.* Washington, D.C.: U.S. Government Printing Office, 1988.

Utian, W. "Oral Contraceptives: Safe After 40?" *Patient Care*, March 30, 1989.

Van Look, P. F. "Postcoital Contraception." *Outlook* 8, no. 3 (September 1990): 2–6.

Vessey, M. P., M. Lawless, et al. "Progestogen-Only Oral Contraception: Findings in a Large Prospective Study with Special Reference to Effectiveness." *British Journal of Family Planning 1985* 10: 117–21.

Vessey, M. P., N. H. Wright, et al. "Fertility After Stopping Different Methods of Contraception." *British Medical Journal*, February 4, 1978.

Weil, M., and T. L. MacDonald. *Fertility Awareness: Natural Birth Control for Women.* Iowa City, Iowa: Emma Goldman Clinic for Women, 1982.

"Which Drugs Truly Interfere with the Efficacy of OCs?" *Contraceptive Technology Update* 10, no. 8 (August 1989): 105–108.

"Which Patients May Benefit from Alternative Contraceptive Methods?" *Contraception Report* 1, no. 4: 7–12.

WHO Special Programme of Research, Development and Research Training in Human Reproduction. "A Randomized, Double-Blind Study of Two Combined and Two Progestogen-Only Contraceptives." *Contraception* 25, no. 3 (March 1982): 243–52.

"Who Will Provide Abortions?" Report of a national symposium sponsored by the National Abortion Federation and the

American College of Obstetricians and Gynecologists. Washington, D. C.: National Abortion Federation, 1990.

Winikoff, B. "Breastfeeding." *Current Opinion in Obstetrics and Gynecology 1990* 2: 548–55.

Winikoff, B., P. Semeraro, and M. Zimmerman. *Contraception During Breastfeeding.* New York: Population Council, 1989.

Wolinsky, H. "U.S. 'Abortion Rights' Threatened by Personnel Shortages." *Medical Post*, May 21, 1991, p. 37.

Wymelenberg, S., for the Institute of Medicine. *Science and Babies: Private Decisions, Public Dilemmas.* Washington, D.C.: National Academy Press, 1990.

Index